CLEAR
THROAT
LIFE

the prescription-free natural
end to post nasal drip

MICHAEL KORTBUS, MD

THE CLEAR THROAT LIFE

THE PRESCRIPTION-FREE NATURAL END TO POST NASAL DRIP

MICHAEL KORTBUS, MD

FIRST EDITION, 2023

PROLOGUE

This book is dedicated to my wife and children who have stood by me and helped me throughout my journey.

I am also grateful to the many patients who have trusted me and shared their stories and concerns, making me a better doctor and clinician along the way. Thank you to the friends and family who gave me advice.

Lastly, I stand on the shoulders of giants – thank you to my mentors and colleagues, as well as my current faculty partners. And thank you to Pexels for providing images.

CONTENTS

SECTION I

INTRODUCTION

1

INTRODUCTION & ACRONYMS

I magine having postnasal drip and throat clearing. Then hoping it goes away. Then seeing a health care worker, maybe at an urgent care center because the time that you become fed up with this is not during regular office hours, or that your primary care office does not have an opening for weeks. But you are ready now!

You speak about your issue, and they wonder if your throat clearing is FROM postnasal drip. They reassure you that all is well, and recommend allergy medicine. The medicine is over the counter, so you are to find it and hope for the best. There is no prescription. After trying this and that medicine – pills, decongestants, pills for mucus, nasal sprays – nothing improves.

You go back to the urgent care or maybe even to primary care who you have waited for an appointment with for weeks. And they reassure you also. They advise that all is well and maybe even give you a prescription. But that doesn't work either. You make an appointment with a specialist or two that have other tools to examine you with, and no progress is made. The post-nasal drip, throat clearing, mucus or phlegm in the throat, cough, voice crackling, sore throat, sense that the throat may close, feeling of a scratch or tickle in the throat, feeling of a lump in the throat, tight swallowing, food feeling like it is "going down the wrong pipe" and more do not let up. **THIS BOOK IS FOR YOU**.

In this book, you will learn about postnasal drip (PND), including its possible causes, symptoms that can go along with it, and non-medical treatments.

You will learn how to free yourself from postnasal drip. My goal is to share my knowledge of helping people overcome postnasal drip to live a clear throat life.

The first section is an introduction.

The second section of the book is dedicated to chemicals, food and behaviors that you have to pay attention to, stop & take care of since you are serious about the clear throat life.

The third section is about lifestyle modifications to get rid of that throat phlegm for good.

The fourth section is about OTC medicines and the last chapter is about miscellaneous concepts related to some who have postnasal drip, throat clearing, mucus or phlegm in the throat, cough, voice crackling, sore throat, sense that the throat may close, feeling of a scratch or tickle in the throat, feeling of a lump in the throat, tight swallowing, food feeling like it is "going down the wrong pipe" and more.

If you are ready to say goodbye to postnasal drip for good, then I encourage you to read on.

First, here is a list of acronyms that will be used:

PND Post nasal drip, or postnasal drip.
PFA BPepsin, foodstuff, acid and bile.
ENT Ear, nose and throat, the initials used for otolaryngologists.
LES Lower esophageal sphincter.
UES Upper esophageal sphincter.
OTC Over-the-counter.
EGD Esophagogastroduodenoscopy, or "endoscopy".
Foodstuff Anything that one puts in the mouth and swallows (e.g. food and drink).
TSL Throat symptom list = postnasal drip,

throat clearing, mucus or phlegm in the throat, cough, voice crackling, sore throat, sense that the throat may close, feeling of a scratch or tickle in the throat, feeling of a lump in the throat, tight swallowing, food feeling like it is "going down the wrong pipe" and more in some (e.g. throwing up, regurgitation, heartburn / pyrosis, etc.).

HCW Health Care Worker.

CTL Clear Throat Life

NB – Note well: Most HCW do not enjoy acronyms (abbreviations) any more than you do. But when they are written so often, many times a day, they serve a purpose!

Also, I want you to know what they mean so that you are equipped to understand things written about PND along the journey of the clear throat life.

2

THE PAIN POINTS OF POSTNASAL DRIP

Postnasal drip is a common medical symptom that can come with a variety of uncomfortable symptoms, including throat clearing, mucus or phlegm in the throat, cough, voice crackling, sore throat, sense that the throat may close, feeling of a scratch or tickle in the throat, feeling of a lump in the throat, tight swallowing, food feeling like it is "going down the wrong pipe" and more. While postnasal drip can be caused by a number of factors, including allergies and the common cold, **CHRONIC postnasal drip is most often caused by reflux.**

This statement that **CHRONIC postnasal drip is most often caused by reflux** is an absolute revelation in and of itself. Please stop here for a moment and really think about that: we are not talking about the nose, sinuses, allergies, and such!

If you have postnasal drip, you know how painful and embarrassing it can be. You may feel like you constantly have to clear your throat, even when there is nothing there. You may also have a cough or a sore throat. And in some cases, postnasal drip can even cause difficulty breathing.

Here are some of the most common pain points of postnasal drip:

- Constant throat clearing: One of the most common side effect of postnasal drip is a constant need to clear your throat. This can be embarrassing and disruptive, especially in social or professional settings.
- Cough: Another common effect of postnasal drip is a cough. This cough can be dry or productive, and it can be difficult to suppress.
- Sore throat: Postnasal drip can also be related to a sore throat. This is because the constant dripping of mucus can irritate the throat lining.
- Difficulty breathing: In some cases, postnasal drip can cause difficulty breathing. This is because the mucus can be in the airway and obstruct.

Again, as one who suffers with postnasal drip, throat clearing, mucus or phlegm in the throat, cough, voice crackling, sore throat, sense that the throat may close, feeling of a scratch or tickle in the throat, feeling of a lump in the throat, tight swallowing, food feeling like it is "going down the wrong pipe" and more, the good news is that there are treatments available that can help. As a master otolaryngologist with more than 20 years' experience helping people, I have seen firsthand the serious effects that postnasal drip can have on people's lives. I have also seen firsthand how effective non-Rx treatments can be in relieving postnasal drip symptoms and improving people's quality of life.

Have you ever felt embarrassed by clearing your throat in public?

Has anybody ever offered you a lozenge because they thought you had a cold?

Do you ever feel like you can't speak in full sentences without having to clear your throat?

If you answered yes to any of these questions, then you are not alone. Millions of people around the world suffer from postnasal drip. But the good news is that there is help available right here in this text.

People seek out what is PND?; how does PND relate to TSL?; is it contagious?; and of course how to get rid of it!

WHAT IS POSTNASAL DRIP?

By now, you might be thinking to yourself "What is the doctor writing about exactly?" I have spent many, many hours breaking down the <u>misnomer</u> that is postnasal drip (PND). Some write the phrase as post nasal drip to break it down and for this next concept, it is helpful to do so. Let us think about these words:

- POST means behind
- NASAL means nose, nasal cavity, sinuses: all that area behind the nostrils
- DRIP means to let fall or be so wet as to shed small drops of liquid

By parsing out these three words, we can see that the phrase itself – Post Nasal Drip – begs the source of the problem! In other words, *Dur! It must be coming from the nose.*

Right? <u>Wrong</u>. After asking many thousands of patients what they mean when they say they have postnasal drip, almost invariably what is meant is that mucus SEEMS to collect in the back of the nose. Or, phlegm in the back / top of the throat. Some will swear they "feel it dripping". The location is behind the "dangling thing", or uvula, some say.

However, PND is a symptom – meaning it is something that you report to the nurse or medical health care worker (HCW).

PND is NOT a sign! PND is not part of the physical examination – which is called a sign in medicine (something we can see, touch, hear or feel during the physical exam.).

If one is examining the throat and notices phlegm or mucus, it is proper to notate "mucus in throat". It would be improper to label this postnasal drip since this PND phrase means it is a symptom and not a sign.

Acute sinusitis of less than a couple of weeks' time – which would be an *acute* (short-lasting) condition and not a *chronic* (perennial, months-long) condition – a health care worker may indeed see mucus draining in the throat. That HCW should not label the chart as

PND unless the patient reports feeling it. Sometimes, mucus is seen in the throat by a dental worker (hygienist, dentist, tech) but they should be noting this as "mucus in the throat". It is important for the medical HCW to know exactly what is being conveyed, otherwise people walking around saying "I have PND" when what they mean is not exactly that.

Less than 5% (five percent) of people complaining of chronic postnasal drip, throat clearing, mucus or phlegm in the throat, cough, voice crackling, sore throat, sense that the throat may close, feeling of a scratch or tickle in the throat, feeling of a lump in the throat, tight swallowing, food feeling like it is "going down the wrong pipe" and more at the office have it from chronic sinusitis.

THE MEDICAL APPROACH TO POSTNASAL DRIP

WHAT IS THE APPROACH TO SOMEONE WITH POSTNASAL DRIP? THE HISTORY.

The approach to the patient with postnasal drip, throat clearing, mucus or phlegm in the throat, cough, voice crackling, sore throat, sense that the throat may close, feeling of a scratch or tickle in the throat, feeling of a lump in the throat, tight swallowing, food feeling like it is "going down the wrong pipe" and more such symptoms begins with a history.

- How long has it been going on?
- Have you seen a HCW about this before?
- Have you tried medicine before?

- Are there other diseases or conditions going on in your life?

And so forth.

What is the approach to someone with postnasal drip? The physical examination.

This is followed by a thorough physical examination including the throat check. Now, sometimes the throat check is performed with a simple [dental] mirror with a long shaft that can look at the throat & larynx (also known as the voice box). However, this requires significant skill and experience – most are not confident with their skill in using this tool.

Therefore, many choose to use a flexible laryngoscope, This is the tool made of fiberoptic glass wires surrounded by a [usually] black plastic sheath that goes through the nose with a light to deliver images to the examiner holding the tool.

However, nearly all otolaryngologists (ENT doctors) do not have an EGD (esophagogastroduodenoscope) to look further at the source of the problem. Therefore it is proper to consider referral to a gastroenterologist (GI doctor) to look further.

Colleagues in medicine can discuss the intricacies of testing, different tools, different subspecialties and more and *that discussion is beyond the scope of this book.* The point is, **you should have a scope that looks at the source of the postnasal drip** which is an EGD with a GI.

WHY NOT JUST PRESCRIBE A MEDICINE?

When I was in training decades ago, we would recommend heavy doses of medicine - most often several times a day - in an effort to resolve PND and the throat symptoms (TSL).

There are several issues that have come up over time and have become more obvious with this approach of "just prescribe a medicine".

First, "just prescribing a medicine" takes away the chance of solving the issue with healthy and natural proactive methods as described in this clear throat life book you now have!

Second, it does solve the HCW dilemma of efficiency in seeing patients, but "just prescribing a medicine" does not delve into remedies that are not pharmaceutical.

Third, many patients simply do not want to take medicine.

Fourth, **medicines used to treat PND are aimed at ACID ONLY!** Medicines prescribed for postnasal drip, throat clearing, mucus or phlegm in the throat, cough, voice crackling, sore throat, sense that the throat may close, feeling of a scratch or tickle in the throat, feeling of a lump in the throat, tight swallowing, food feeling like it is "going down the wrong pipe" and more are ANTACID in nature. *What about bile, pepsin and foodstuff?*

Fifth, medicines have copays and usually cost more than other remedies, especially the free remedies you are learning about in this CTL book.

Sixth, when a person stops taking antacids, they can have "rebound" symptoms (see TSL) and severe throat pain with heartburn (aka pyrosis) what was worse than when they started.

Seventh, if you "just take medicine" and you get better that is wonderful, but how and when do you stop? This is – or should be – a careful process with your HCW due to point six in the previous sentence.

Eighth, if a HCW "just prescribes a medicine" and it does not work, it DOES NOT MEAN YOU DO NOT HAVE reflux as the cause for throat symptoms. It only means that it is more likely to be from foodstuff, bile, pepsin, or some other anatomical or behavioral reason and NOT ACID.

THE CLEAR THROAT LIFE | 27

When I examine a patient and determine that they have the symptom of postnasal drip and start educating about reflux, many automatically ask "Oh, you mean acid reflux?". And I always say it is better to use the one word. This helps you understand that there are other causes that are not addressed with "just prescribing a medicine".

Ninth, many of the medicines used to treat PND & TSL can cause electrolyte deficiencies, have been linked to increased chance for pneumonia, colitis, hip fracture and even dementia.

I will stop this list here – this would be enough for most to avoid medicine for reflux & PND.

However, there are still many patients who need to take such medicine for throat symptoms – again, have a conversation with your HCW, pharmacist, nurse or advanced care provider to see if they are right for you.

Your HCW may insist that you stay on medicine. Follow their advice. But do not believe that a negative barium swallow or barium esophagram is sufficient to tell you there is no reflux. It simply does not have the statistical strength to do so. Likewise, a negative Bravo probe is not going to tell you there is no reflux since it only measures – you guessed it – acid!

Interestingly, when I am getting to know a patient and make the connection between postnasal drip and reflux, the first thing many people say is "Oh, you mean acid reflux?" Immediately, no. I have to use this time to educate the person right there – because reflux is not all about acid and taking acid medicine is not the answer for many.

SECTION II

STOP

5

STOP THESE THINGS!

Certain foods and some drinks that we consume cause the feeling and the symptom of postnasal drip. And some food and drinks can make pre-existing postnasal drip worse.

This section of the CTL book will go through food, dink, and behavior that causes PND and TSL. For example, drinking coffee, eating spicy foods and/or smoking cigarettes will cause postnasal drip, throat clearing, mucus or phlegm in the throat, cough, voice crackling, sore throat, sense that the throat may close, feeling of a scratch or tickle in the throat, feeling of a lump in the throat, tight swallowing, food feeling like it is "going down the wrong pipe" and more for many people.

When reading this section, <u>you will notice repetition</u> of certain concepts and phrases. Please know this is intentional. I have kept this this way for two reasons:

A) So that if someone uses this as a reference, as it is intended, they can pick up this book, head to the chapter and see the words and ideas spelled out, rather than having to bounce around seeking out reasons elsewhere.

B) To show you that there are only a limited – very limited – number of ways that "things" (food, drink, smoking, etc.) affect the body, believe it or not.

Truth be told, health science is an evolving science so I write this book mindfully - knowing that as time and research progress, a greater understanding of the things that affect us and create symptoms will be known. Look forward to another edition at that time!

I also hope for us to research and understand exactly how we become affected by our environment on a granular / cellular level so that better therapies can become known and safely used. And this knowledge will also look at how "the things" interact with each other within us.

6

TOBACCO, NICOTINE, &
MARIJUANA

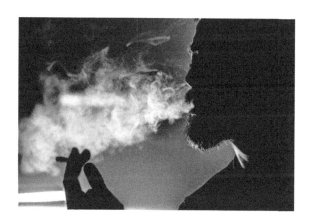

TOBACCO AND NICOTINE

Interesting that tobacco was chosen as the first chapter of the book to focus on PND, right? Smoker or not, *do not skip this chapter!* Many believe that it was through tobacco use that the relationship between PND and reflux came to be known.

Most people – but definitely family members & HCW - are glad to know that the rate of tobacco and nicotine use is down, since there are so many direct and indirect effects of using nicotine. But early studies proved that nicotine has many deleterious effects to the throat (see below) and that for those who do not use nicotine, the degree to which postnasal drip, throat clearing, mucus or phlegm in the throat, cough, voice crackling, sore throat, sense that the throat may close, feeling of a scratch or tickle in the throat, feeling of a lump in the throat, tight swallowing, food feeling like it is "going down the wrong pipe" and more begin after using nicotine is remarkable.

I do not recommend trying nicotine if you don't ever use it, but for those who take up using nicotine in any way, the degree to which it irritates the throat and causes the list of throat symptoms (TSL) is remarkable.

Tobacco, nicotine, marijuana, and other products - smoked, chewed, or exposed to - can make postnasal drip worse via stimulation of reflux in a number of ways.

First, nicotine relaxes the lower esophageal sphincter (LES). The LES is a muscle valve that separates the stomach from the esophagus. When the LES is relaxed, then pepsin, foodstuff, acid, and bile (PFAB) from the stomach can return back up into the throat, causing reflux.

Second, tobacco and marijuana can irritate the lining of the throat, making it more sensitive to pepsin, food-stuff, acid and bile reflux.

Third, tobacco and marijuana can increase production of stomach acid.

Fourth, tobacco and marijuana can slow down the movement of food through the digestive system. This can give pepsin, foodstuff, acid and bile more time to back up into the throat.

THE EFFECTS OF NICOTINE ON POSTNASAL DRIP

Nicotine is a highly addictive substance that is found in tobacco products, including cigarettes, vapes, cigars, and chewing tobacco. It is also found in some electronic cigarettes and nicotine replacement therapies (NRTs), such as gum and patches.

Nicotine has a number of effects on the body, including:

- Relaxing the LES
- Increasing stomach acid production
- Slowing down the movement of food through the digestive system
- Irritating the lining of the esophagus & throat

All of these effects contribute to postnasal drip, throat clearing, mucus or phlegm in the throat, cough, voice crackling, sore throat, sense that the throat may close, feeling of a scratch or tickle in the throat, feeling of a lump in the throat, tight swallowing, food feeling like it is "going down the wrong pipe" and more.

MARIJUANA AND CANNABIDIOL (CBD)

The relaxation of marijuana law across many regions has led to a rise in marijuana and CBD usage. Therefore, HCW are seeing more who have postnasal drip, throat clearing, mucus or phlegm in the throat, cough, voice crackling, sore throat, sense that the throat may close, feeling of a scratch or tickle in the throat, feeling of a lump in the throat, tight swallowing, food feeling like it is "going down the wrong pipe" and more. After ruling other issues out, it can be marijuana use that is the culprit. When many stop using CBD or MJ, the drip resolves as well.

Marijuana smoke contains a number of harmful chemicals, including cannabinoids. Cannabinoids are the compounds in marijuana that produce its psychoactive effects.

Cannabinoids have a number of effects on the body, including:

- Relaxing the LES
- Irritating the lining of the throat

These effects can contribute to postnasal drip.

If you have postnasal drip, the first way to reduce your risk of symptoms is to avoid the products that can make it worse. This includes tobacco, nicotine, marijuana, and more that you will be learning about in this clear throat life book.

If you are a smoker, quitting is the best thing you can do for your health. Quitting smoking will help reduce your risk of postnasal drip.

If you use nicotine replacement therapy (NRT), you may want to talk to your doctor about switching to a different type of NRT. Some types of NRT, such as gum and patches, can still irritate the lining of the throat and make PND and throat symptoms.

7

LYING DOWN

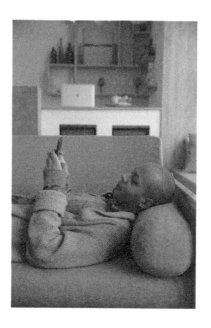

When you eat a meal, the stomach produces substances to help break down the food.

These substances or chemicals made by your own body are normally kept in the stomach by the lower esophageal sphincter (LES). The LES is a muscle valve that separates the stomach from the esophagus.

When I say lying down, I am purposefully not saying going to bed. Many have a meal then lie down with a laptop or smartphone, watch TV, watch their kids from a lying position, read a book while lying down, and more. It is the act of making the torso (chest) parallel to the ground and horizontal that allows PFAB (Pepsin, foodstuff, acid and bile) to come up into the throat.

However, when you lie down after eating, the LES can relax and allow PFAB to back up into the throat. This can cause a number of uncomfortable symptoms, such as heartburn, chest pain, and regurgitation. Also, and most importantly, lying down after eating is a common and direct culprit for postnasal drip, throat clearing, mucus or phlegm in the throat, cough, voice crackling, sore throat, sense that the throat may close, feeling of a scratch or tickle in the throat, feeling of a lump in the throat, tight swallowing, food feeling like it is "going down the wrong pipe" and more.

Here are some of the reasons why eating a meal and then lying down can cause reflux:

- Gravity: When you lie down, the stomach is at the same level as the throat. This makes it easier for pepsin, foodstuff, acid and bile to back up into the throat.
- Relaxation of the LES: Lying down can relax the LES, which allows pepsin, foodstuff, acid and bile to back up into the throat.
- Increased pressure in the stomach: Lying down can increase the pressure in the stomach, which can also push pepsin, foodstuff, acid and bile back up into the throat.

HOW TO REDUCE THE RISK OF REFLUX AFTER EATING

If you are prone to reflux, there are a number of things you can do to reduce your risk of symptoms after eating:

- Wait to lie down: After eating, wait at least three hours before lying down. This will give your stomach time to empty and reduce the amount of pepsin, foodstuff, acid and bile that can back up into the throat.

- Elevate your torso: If you need to lie down after eating, elevate your head by six to eight inches. This will help to keep the pepsin, foodstuff, acid and bile below the level of the throat. Consider a bed rest.

- Eat smaller meals: Eating smaller meals will help to reduce the pressure in the stomach and make it less likely that pepsin, foodstuff, acid and bile will back up into the throat.

- Avoid certain foods and drinks: There are a number of foods and drinks discussed through this book that can trigger PND, such as caffeine, alcohol, fatty foods, and spicy foods. Avoid these foods and drinks after eating to reduce your risk of symptoms.

8

FOODS TO AVOID

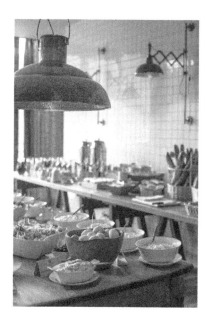

F atty foods, fried foods, and other heavy foods can cause postnasal drip and reflux into the throat in a number of ways.

First, fatty foods and fried foods are more difficult to digest than other foods. This means that they stay in the stomach for a longer period of time. The longer food stays in the stomach, the more time it has to produce PFAB (Pepsin, foodstuff, acid and bile). This increased Pepsin, foodstuff, acid and bile production can lead to reflux.

Second, fatty foods and fried foods can relax the lower esophageal sphincter (LES). The LES is a muscle valve that separates the stomach from the throat. When the LES is relaxed, acid and bile from the stomach can back up into the throat, causing PND.

Third, heavy foods can increase pressure in the stomach. This increased pressure can push pepsin, foodstuff, acid and bile back up into the throat, causing postnasal drip, throat clearing, mucus or phlegm in the throat, cough, voice crackling, sore throat, sense that the throat may close, feeling of a scratch or tickle in the throat, feeling of a lump in the throat, tight swallowing, food feeling like it is "going down the wrong pipe" and more..

In addition to these three main ways, fatty foods, fried foods, and other heavy foods can also cause reflux by:

- Stimulating the production of gastrin, a hormone that increases stomach acid production.
- Delaying gastric emptying, which is the process of food moving from the stomach into the small intestine.
- Irritating the lining of the throat, making it more sensitive to pepsin, foodstuff, acid and bile reflux.

Here are some examples of fatty foods, fried foods, and other heavy foods that can trigger reflux:

- Fatty meats, such as bacon, sausage, and marbled beef
- Fatty foods: butter, cream, cheese, whole milk, ice cream, fatty meats, bacon, sausage, fried chicken, fries, potato chips, onion rings, pizza, hamburgers, hot dogs, gravy, pastries, cookies, cakes
- Fried foods, such as fries, onion rings, and chicken nuggets
- Full-fat dairy products, such as cream, cheese, and butter

If you have PND, it is important to avoid or limit your intake of fatty foods, fried foods, and other heavy foods. You may also want to keep a food diary to track which foods trigger your reflux symptoms. In other words, track the time you eat the food then the onset of the symptom.

Remember the TSL: Throat symptom list includes but is not limited to postnasal drip, throat clearing, mucus or phlegm in the throat, cough, voice crackling, sore throat, sense that the throat may close, feeling of a scratch or tickle in the throat, feeling of a lump in the throat, tight swallowing, food feeling like it is "going down the wrong pipe" and more.

At times, a person can pinpoint one very specific trigger and live the clear throat life after avoiding that one trigger!

HOW TO REDUCE THE RISK OF PND CAUSED BY FATTY FOODS, FRIED FOODS, AND OTHER HEAVY FOODS

Here are some tips for reducing the risk of PND caused by fatty foods, fried foods, and other heavy foods. If you are prone to postnasal drip, throat clearing, mucus or phlegm in the throat, cough, voice crackling, sore throat, sense that the throat may close, feeling of a scratch or tickle in the throat, feeling of a lump in the throat, tight swallowing, food feeling like it is "going down the wrong pipe" and more, there are a number of things you can do to reduce your risk of symptoms after eating fatty foods, fried foods, and other heavy foods:

- Avoid or limit your intake of these foods: The best way to reduce the risk of reflux is to avoid or limit your intake of fatty foods, fried foods, and other heavy foods.
- Eat smaller meals: Eating smaller meals will help to reduce the pressure in the stomach and make it less likely that pepsin, foodstuff, acid and bile will back up into the throat.
- Avoid eating late at night: Eating late at night can give pepsin, foodstuff, acid and bile less time to digest before you go to bed. This can increase your risk of reflux.
- Avoid lying down after eating.
- Elevate your head when you sleep: Elevating your head by six to eight inches can help to keep pepsin, foodstuff, acid and bile below the level of the throat.
- Avoid alcohol, caffeine, and carbonated beverages: Alcohol and caffeine can relax the

LES and increase the production of pepsin, acid and bile.

- Lose weight if you are overweight or obese: Obesity can increase the pressure in the stomach and make it.
- Quit smoking (see chapter 6 above).
- Follow the other clear throat life sections in this book!

9

ALCOHOL, CHOCOLATE, AND SOFT DRINKS

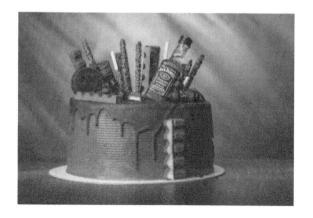

A lcohol, chocolate, and soft drinks (including fruit juice, carbonated beverages, sodas, and seltzer) are all common triggers of postnasal drip, throat clearing, mucus or phlegm in the throat, cough, voice crackling, sore throat, sense that the throat may close, feeling of a scratch or tickle in the throat, feeling of a lump in the throat, tight swallowing, food feeling like it is "going down the wrong pipe" and more.

ALCOHOL

Alcohol relaxes the lower esophageal sphincter (LES). The LES is a muscle valve that separates the stomach from the throat. When the LES is relaxed, pepsin, foodstuff, acid and bile from the stomach can back up into the throat, causing reflux.

Alcohol also increases the production of stomach acid. This increased acid production can contribute to throat reflux.

Alcohol irritates the lining of the throat, making it more sensitive to pepsin, foodstuff, acid and bile reflux.

CHOCOLATE

Chocolate contains caffeine, which can relax the LES and increase stomach acid production.

Chocolate contains fat, which can delay gastric emptying and increase pressure in the stomach, both of which can contribute to reflux.

Chocolate contains methylxanthines (caffeine and theobromine), which are compounds that can relax the

LES and increase stomach acid production. Methylxan-thines are also found in coffee, tea, and energy drinks. Caffeine is a form of methylxanthine.

SOFT DRINKS

Soft drinks, including fruit juice, carbonated beverages, sodas, and seltzer, can all trigger throat reflux for a number of reasons.

- Carbonation: The carbonation in soft drinks can irritate the lining of the throat and make it more sensitive to pepsin, foodstuff, acid and bile. Also, carbonation in sparkling water, which typically has no calories, is made when carbon dioxide gas is dissolved in plain water, a process known as carbonation. This results not only in the bubbles many are seeking, but also creates carbonic acid, which gives fizzy water a mildly tart flavor.
- Sugar: The high sugar content in soft drinks can delay gastric emptying, which is the process of food moving from the stomach into the small intestine. This delay can give pepsin, foodstuff, acid and bile more time to back up into the throat.

- Caffeine: The caffeine in soft drinks can relax the LES and increase stomach acid production.

In addition to the above, here are some other reasons why you should avoid alcohol, chocolate, and soft drinks if you have postnasal drip, throat clearing, mucus or phlegm in the throat, cough, voice crackling, sore throat, sense that the throat may close, feeling of a scratch or tickle in the throat, feeling of a lump in the throat, tight swallowing, food feeling like it is "going down the wrong pipe" and more:

- Alcohol can dehydrate you. Dehydration can make throat reflux worse.
- Chocolate can be high in fat. Fatty foods can relax the LES and increase stomach acid production (see Chapter 8 above).
- Soft drinks can be acidic. Acidic drinks can irritate the lining of the throat and make it more sensitive to pepsin, foodstuff, acid and bile reflux.

If you have PND, it is important to avoid or limit your intake of alcohol, chocolate, and soft drinks. This will help to reduce your risk of symptoms.

Here are some tips for avoiding alcohol, chocolate, and soft drinks:

- Choose water or other unsweetened beverages instead of soft drinks.
- Limit your intake of alcoholic beverages.
- Avoid eating chocolate, especially if it contains caffeine.
- If you do choose to eat chocolate, eat it in moderation and choose dark chocolate over milk chocolate.

10

COFFEE AND TEA

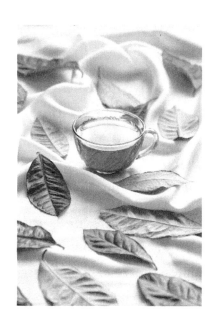

Coffee is a popular beverage enjoyed by people all over the world. In fact, even for many HCW it is so prominent, it might as well be its own food group!

For many, stopping coffee and/or tea is a no-go, a deal-breaker, and there is "no way" they can do it.

However, for people with postnasal drip, throat clearing, mucus or phlegm in the throat, cough, voice crackling, sore throat, sense that the throat may close, feeling of a scratch or tickle in the throat, feeling of a lump in the throat, tight swallowing, food feeling like it is "going down the wrong pipe" and more, **coffee can be THE problem**.

Caffeine, the main active ingredient in coffee, can relax the lower esophageal sphincter (LES), which is the muscle valve that separates the stomach from the esophagus. When the LES is relaxed, acid and bile from the stomach can back up into the throat, causing reflux.

In addition to relaxing the LES, caffeine can also increase stomach acid production. This is because caffeine stimulates the release of gastrin, a hormone that tells the stomach to produce acid.

In addition to its effects on the LES and stomach acid production, coffee can also irritate the lining of the throat by itself. This can make the throat more sensitive to pepsin, foodstuff, acid and bile reflux.

SCIENTIFIC EVIDENCE OF THE CONNECTION BETWEEN COFFEE AND PND

There is a growing body of scientific evidence that supports the link between coffee, postnasal drip and throat symptoms. There was a state-of-the-art review in the journal Nutrients in 2022 that can be accessed for free online [Nehlig A. Effects of Coffee on the Gastro-Intestinal Tract: A Narrative Review and Literature Update. Nutrients. 2022 Jan 17;14(2):399. doi: 10.3390/nu14020399. PMID: 35057580; PMCID: PMC8778943.]

How to reduce the risk of reflux caused by coffee

If you have PND and you want to continue drinking coffee, there are a few things you can do to reduce the risk of the TSL symptoms:

- Limit your intake of coffee to one or two cups per day.
- Avoid drinking coffee on an empty stomach.
- Drink coffee with food or after a meal.
- Choose decaf coffee over regular coffee.

- Add milk but not high fat cream (see chapter 8 above) to your coffee to help buffer the acidity.

Be mindful while stopping caffeine, however. If you have used caffeinated products daily for many years, it can cause a serious headache and other symptoms. Please have your HCW assist in caffeine management.

11

CITRUS

INTRODUCTION

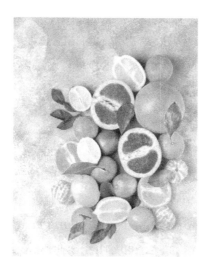

Citrus fruits, such as oranges, grapefruits, lemons, and limes, are a popular and healthy snack. Citrus fruits are renowned for their high vitamin C content and refreshing flavor. However, their acidic nature can play a significant role in worsening postnasal drip. Understanding the mechanisms behind this effect is important for individuals managing PND and making informed dietary choices. For people with postnasal drip, citrus fruits can be a trigger that worsens symptoms. In this chapter, we will discuss in depth exactly how and why citrus fruits can make throat reflux worse. We will also provide some tips for avoiding citrus fruits or reducing their impact on your symptoms.

HOW CITRUS FRUITS CAN MAKE PND & THROAT REFLUX WORSE

There are several reasons why citrus fruits can make throat reflux worse.

- Citrus fruits are acidic. The acidity in citrus fruits can irritate the lining of the throat and make it more sensitive to stomach acid.
- Citrus fruits can relax the lower esophageal sphincter (LES). The LES is a muscle valve that separates the stomach from the throat. When the LES is relaxed, it is more likely to open and allow stomach acid to back up into the throat.

- Citrus fruits can increase stomach acid production. Eating citrus fruits can stimulate the stomach to produce more acid. This can lead to an increase in the amount of stomach acid in the throat, which can worsen reflux symptoms.
- Direct Irritation of the Throat Lining: The acidic nature of citrus juices and fruits can directly irritate the delicate lining of the throat, causing inflammation and exacerbating reflux symptoms.

INDIVIDUAL SENSITIVITY

It is important to note that individual sensitivity to citrus fruits varies. While some individuals may experience significant postnasal drip and TSL after consuming citrus fruits, others may have little or no reaction. This variability is likely influenced by factors such as the severity of symptoms, the type and amount of citrus fruit consumed, and individual susceptibility to PFAB (pepsin, foodstuff, acid and bile).

Managing Reflux with Dietary Modifications

For individuals with reflux, managing citrus intake can be a helpful dietary strategy. However, it is crucial to approach this with caution and personalization. Avoiding citrus fruits altogether may not be necessary for everyone. Instead, individuals can experiment with different amounts and types of citrus fruits to determine their personal tolerance level.

Tips for Avoiding Citrus Fruits or Reducing Their Impact on Your Symptoms

If you have postnasal drip, there are a few things you can do to avoid citrus fruits or reduce their impact on your symptoms:

- Eliminate citrus fruits from your diet. This is the most effective way to avoid the trigger.
- Eat citrus fruits in moderation. If you must eat citrus fruits, eat them in moderation and avoid eating them before bed.
- Choose less acidic citrus fruits. Grapefruits are the most acidic citrus fruit, so choose oranges, lemons, or limes instead.
- Cook citrus fruits. Cooking citrus fruits can reduce their acidity.
- Eat citrus fruits with other foods. Eating citrus fruits with other foods can help to buffer the acidity.

Citrus fruits can make throat reflux worse by irritating the lining of the throat, relaxing the LES, and increasing stomach acid production. If you have throat reflux, it is important to be aware of the symptoms and triggers. There are a few things you can do to avoid citrus fruits or reduce their impact on your symptoms.

12

DAIRY

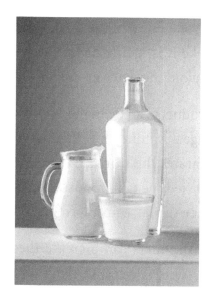

WHAT IS THE DAIRY GROUP?

The dairy group is a food group that includes milk, yogurt, cheese, lactose-free milk, and fortified soy milk and yogurt. Dairy products can be a good source of protein, calcium, and other nutrients.

Why should people with PND avoid the dairy group?

There are a few reasons why people with postnasal drip, throat clearing, mucus or phlegm in the throat, cough, voice crackling, sore throat, sense that the throat may close, feeling of a scratch or tickle in the throat, feeling of a lump in the throat, tight swallowing, food feeling like it is "going down the wrong pipe" and more should avoid the dairy group.

First, dairy products can be high in fat. Fat can relax the lower esophageal sphincter (LES), which is a muscle valve that separates the stomach from the throat. When the LES is relaxed, pepsin, foodstuff, acid and bile can back up into the throat, causing reflux.

Second, dairy products can increase the production of stomach acid. This is because dairy products contain calcium, which is a mineral that stimulates the stomach to produce acid. Calcium can also relax the LES. Dairy products are a good source of calcium, so people who consume a lot of dairy may be more likely to experience reflux.

Third, dairy products can irritate the lining of the throat. This can make the throat more sensitive to Pepsin, foodstuff, acid and bile.

Also, dairy products can contain casein, a protein that can thicken mucus. This thickened mucus can be more difficult to clear from the throat and can make reflux symptoms worse.

What is the link between lactose intolerance and reflux?

Lactose intolerance is a condition in which people have difficulty digesting lactose, a sugar found in milk and other dairy products. When people with lactose intolerance eat dairy products, they can experience a variety of symptoms, including gas, bloating, diarrhea, and abdominal cramps.

Some people with lactose intolerance also experience reflux after eating dairy products. This is because lactose intolerance can cause inflammation in the intestines. This inflammation can lead to an increase in stomach acid production and relaxation of the LES.

WHAT ARE SOME DAIRY-FREE ALTERNATIVES THAT PEOPLE WITH REFLUX CAN ENJOY?

There are a number of dairy-free alternatives that people with reflux can enjoy. These include:

- Plant-based milks, such as almond milk, soy milk, and oat milk
- Plant-based yogurts, such as almond yogurt, soy yogurt, and coconut yogurt
- Plant-based cheeses, such as almond cheese, soy cheese, and cashew cheese
- Lactose-free dairy products, such as lactose-free milk, lactose-free yogurt, and lactose-free cheese

TIPS FOR AVOIDING DAIRY PRODUCTS

Here are some tips for avoiding dairy products, If you have postnasal drip, throat clearing, mucus or phlegm in the throat, cough, voice crackling, sore throat, sense that the throat may close, feeling of a scratch or tickle in the throat, feeling of a lump in the throat, tight swallowing, food feeling like it is "going down the wrong pipe" and more and you want to continue eating dairy products, there are a few things you can do to reduce the risk of reflux symptoms:

- Choose low-fat or fat-free dairy products.
- Avoid hard cheeses, such as cheddar and Swiss, as they are high in fat and casein.
- Choose soft cheeses, such as mozzarella and ricotta, as they are lower in fat and casein.
- Avoid yogurt that contains added sugar or fruit.
- Fortified soy milk and yogurt are good alternatives to dairy products for people with reflux.
- Read food labels carefully to check for dairy ingredients.
- Look for dairy-free alternatives to your favorite foods.
- Ask about dairy-free options when eating out.
- Keep a food diary to track which foods trigger your reflux symptoms.

Several studies suggest that people with PND may benefit from avoiding dairy products, or at least switching to lactose-free dairy products.

If you are considering eliminating dairy products from your diet, it is important to talk to your doctor to make sure that you are getting all the nutrients you need.

13

PEANUTS AND PEANUT DERIVATIVES

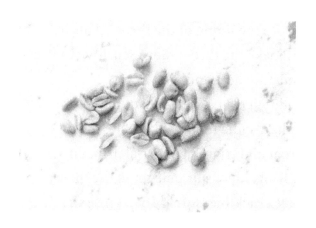

P eanuts and peanut derivatives, such as peanut butter, are common triggers of reflux. There are a few reasons for this:

- Fat: Peanuts and peanut butter are high in fat. Fat can relax the lower esophageal sphincter

(LES), which is the muscle valve that separates the stomach from the throat. When the LES is relaxed, pepsin, foodstuff, acid and bile can back up into the throat, causing reflux.

- Allergy: Peanuts are one of the most common food allergens. If you have a peanut allergy, eating peanuts or peanut butter can trigger an allergic reaction. This reaction can cause inflammation of the throat, which can lead to reflux.

- Tannins: Peanuts and peanut butter contain tannins. Tannins are compounds that can irritate the lining of the throat. This irritation can make the throat more sensitive to Pepsin, foodstuff, acid and bile.

- Acidity: Peanuts and peanut butter are also acidic. Acidic foods can irritate the lining of the throat and trigger postnasal drip, throat clearing, mucus or phlegm in the throat, cough, voice crackling, sore throat, sense that the throat may close, feeling of a scratch or tickle in the throat, feeling of a lump in the throat, tight swallowing, food feeling like it is "going down the wrong pipe" and more..

SYMPTOMS OF REFLUX TRIGGERED BY PEANUTS OR PEANUT BUTTER

The symptoms of reflux triggered by peanuts or peanut butter are the same as the symptoms of reflux caused by other foods. These symptoms can include postnasal drip, throat clearing, mucus or phlegm in the throat, cough, voice crackling, sore throat, sense that the throat may close, feeling of a scratch or tickle in the throat, feeling of a lump in the throat, tight swallowing, food feeling like it is "going down the wrong pipe" and more:

- Heartburn
- Chest pain
- Regurgitation
- Sour taste in the mouth
- Difficulty swallowing
- Wheezing

HOW TO REDUCE THE RISK OF PND TRIGGERED BY PEANUTS OR PEANUT BUTTER

If you have postnasal drip, throat clearing, mucus or phlegm in the throat, cough, voice crackling, sore throat, sense that the throat may close, feeling of a scratch or tickle in the throat, feeling of a lump in the throat, tight swallowing, food feeling like it is "going down the wrong pipe" and more, it is best to avoid peanuts and peanut derivatives altogether. However, if you do choose to eat peanuts or peanut butter, there are a few things you can do to reduce the risk of reflux:

- Eat peanuts or peanut butter in moderation.
- Eat peanuts or peanut butter with a meal. This can help to slow down digestion and reduce the amount of pepsin, foodstuff, acid and bile that backs up into the throat.
- Avoid lying down after eating peanuts or peanut butter.

14

SUGAR AND SUGAR DERIVATIVES

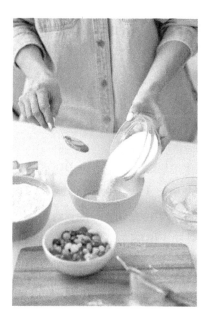

S ugar and sugar derivatives, such as syrup, can trigger postnasal drip in a number of ways.

First, sugar and sugar derivatives can relax the lower esophageal sphincter (LES). The LES is a muscle valve that separates the stomach from the throat. When the LES is relaxed, pepsin, foodstuff, acid and bile can back up into the throat, causing reflux.

Second, sugar and sugar derivatives can increase stomach acid production. This is because sugar stimulates the release of gastrin, a hormone that tells the stomach to produce acid.

Third, sugar and sugar derivatives can delay gastric emptying. Gastric emptying is the process of food moving from the stomach into the small intestine. When gastric emptying is delayed, food stays in the stomach for a longer period of time, which gives pepsin, foodstuff, acid and bile more time to back up into the throat.

Fourth, and perhaps most importantly, sugar can DIRECTLY irritate the lining of the throat. This can make the throat more sensitive to stomach pepsin, foodstuff, acid and bile, increasing the risk of postnasal drip, throat clearing, mucus or phlegm in the throat, cough, voice crackling, sore throat, sense that the throat may close, feeling of a scratch or tickle in the throat, feeling of a lump in the throat, tight swallowing, food feeling like it is "going down the wrong pipe" and more.

In addition to these four main ways, sugar and sugar derivatives can also trigger reflux by:

- Promoting the growth of harmful bacteria in the stomach, which can produce toxins that contribute to inflammation and irritation of the lining of the throat.
- Increasing inflammation throughout the body, which can make reflux symptoms worse.

Here are some examples of sugar and sugar derivatives that can trigger reflux:

- Added sugars, such as sucrose (table sugar), fructose (corn syrup), and glucose.
- Natural sugars, such as honey, maple syrup, and agave nectar.
- Syrups, such as high-fructose corn syrup, chocolate syrup, and caramel syrup.
- Soft drinks, including fruit juice.
- Candy, cake & cookies
- Baked goods
- Desserts
- Pastries
- Sugary cereals
- Coffee with sugar
- Tea with sugar

SHOULD I AVOID ALL SUGAR AND SUGAR DERIVATIVES IF I HAVE PND?

It is not necessary to avoid all sugar and sugar derivatives if you have PND. However, you may want to limit your intake of sugary foods and drinks, especially those that are high in fat and/or acidic.

If you are unsure whether sugar or sugar derivatives trigger your postnasal drip, it is a good idea to keep a food diary. This can help you to identify the foods that are most likely to cause your symptoms.

Here are some tips for reducing the risk of reflux caused by sugar and sugar derivatives:

- Avoid or limit your intake of added sugars, natural sugars, and syrups.
- Choose water or unsweetened beverages instead of soft drinks, fruit juice, and sugary drinks.
- Eat whole fruits and vegetables instead of candy and baked goods.
- Cook and prepare your own meals so that you can control the amount of sugar and sugar derivatives that you consume.
- Eat sugary foods and drinks with a meal. This can help to slow down digestion and reduce the

amount of pepsin, foodstuff, acid and bile that backs up into the throat.

- Avoid lying down after eating sugary foods and drinks.

15

PROCESSED FOODS

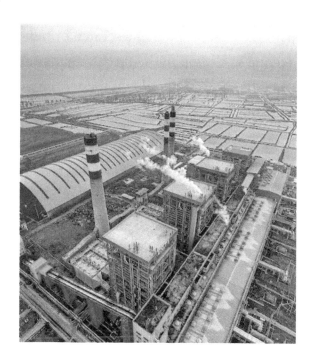

W e have all been to the store and bought some processed foods and marveled at the long lists of ingredients. What are these words? What do they mean? How are they added to the food? How do these ingredients interact with each other? How do they affect my body?

In a sense, going out to eat at some restaurants – typically fast-food restaurants – poses the same list of questions and may come with similar risk of generating postnasal drip, throat clearing, mucus or phlegm in the throat, cough, voice crackling, sore throat, sense that the throat may close, feeling of a scratch or tickle in the throat, feeling of a lump in the throat, tight swallowing, food feeling like it is "going down the wrong pipe" and more.

Processed foods are foods that have been altered from their natural state through methods such as canning, freezing, drying, or smoking. Processed food derivatives are foods that are made from processed foods, such as syrup.

Processed foods and processed food derivatives, such as syrup (as also described in chapter 14), can trigger postnasal drip in a number of ways.

First, processed foods are often high in fat and/or acidic. Fat and acid can relax the lower esophageal sphincter (LES), which is the muscle valve that separates the stomach from the throat. When the LES is relaxed, pepsin, foodstuff, acid and bile can back up into the throat, causing reflux.

Second, processed foods often contain added sugar. Sugar can also relax the LES and increase stomach acid production.

Third, processed foods are often difficult to digest. This can cause food to stay in the stomach for a longer period of time, which can increase the risk of reflux.

Fourth, processed foods often contain artificial ingredients, such as preservatives and flavorings. These artificial ingredients can irritate the lining of the throat, making it more sensitive to pepsin, foodstuff, acid and bile.

Which processed foods are most likely to trigger reflux?

Some common processed foods that are likely to trigger reflux include:

- Seed oils (e.g. Canola oil, Vegetable oil)
- Dressings and sauces
- Margarine
- Fast food
- Frozen meals

- Canned foods
- Processed meats (e.g., cold cuts, hot dogs, bacon, sausage)
- Frankenfoods like plant-based meat (ultra-processed food)
- Smoked meats
- Fried foods
- Candy
- Chocolate
- Cookies
- Cakes & baked goods
- Ice cream
- Soda
- Sports drinks
- Juice
- Sweet tea
- Coffee with sugar and cream
- Sugary drinks

Should I avoid all processed foods if I have reflux?

It is not necessary to avoid all processed foods if you have reflux. However, you may want to avoid processed foods that are high in fat, acid, sugar, and/or artificial ingredients. You may also want to limit your intake of other processed foods.

If you are unsure whether processed foods trigger your reflux, it is a good idea to keep a food diary. This can help you to identify the foods that are most likely to cause your symptoms.

Here are some tips for reducing the risk of postnasal drip if you do consume processed foods:

- Choose processed foods that are low in fat, acid, sugar, and/or artificial ingredients.
- Limit your intake of processed foods.
- Eat processed foods with a meal. This can help to slow down digestion and reduce the amount of pepsin, foodstuff, acid and bile that backs up into the throat.
- Avoid lying down after eating processed foods.

16

PEPPERMINT

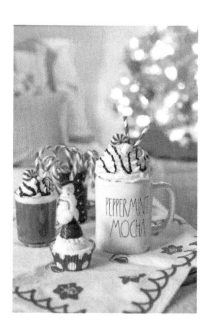

P eppermint is a popular herb that is used in a variety of foods and beverages, including tea, candy, and gum. Peppermint is also used in some medications, such as over-the-counter indigestion remedies.

- Relaxing the lower esophageal sphincter (LES): The LES is a muscle valve that separates the stomach from the throat. When the LES is relaxed, stomach acid can back up into the throat, causing reflux. Peppermint contains menthol, which can relax the LES.
- Increasing stomach acid production: Peppermint can increase stomach acid production by stimulating the release of gastrin, a hormone that tells the stomach to produce acid.
- Irritating the lining of the throat: Peppermint can irritate the lining of the throat, making it more sensitive to reflux.

WHICH PEPPERMINT PRODUCTS ARE MOST LIKELY TO TRIGGER POSTNASAL DRIP?

Peppermint products in all forms can trigger postnasal drip, including:

- Peppermint tea
- Peppermint candy

- Peppermint chewing gum
- Peppermint oil capsules
- Peppermint capsules

SHOULD I AVOID ALL PEPPERMINT PRODUCTS IF I HAVE POSTNASAL DRIP?

It is best to avoid any and all peppermint products if you have postnasal drip, throat clearing, mucus or phlegm in the throat, cough, voice crackling, sore throat, sense that the throat may close, feeling of a scratch or tickle in the throat, feeling of a lump in the throat, tight swallowing, food feeling like it is "going down the wrong pipe" and more.

However, if you do choose to consume peppermint products, it is important to do so in moderation. You may also want to avoid consuming peppermint products before bed, as this can increase the risk of reflux during the night.

If you are unsure whether peppermint triggers your PND, **it is a good idea to keep a food diary**. This can help you to identify the foods that are most likely to cause your symptoms.

How to reduce the risk of reflux caused by peppermint

If you have reflux and you want to continue using peppermint, there are a few things you can do to reduce the risk of reflux:

- Limit your intake of peppermint.
- Avoid peppermint before bed.
- Avoid peppermint if you have a full stomach.
- Take peppermint with food.
- Choose peppermint products that are low in sugar and acidity.

If you have reflux and you are avoiding or limiting your intake of peppermint, you may still need to take medication to control your symptoms. There are a number of medications available that can help to reduce stomach acid production and relieve the symptoms of reflux.

PEPPERMINT AND REFLUX MEDICATION

It is important to note that peppermint can interact with some reflux medications. For example, peppermint can reduce the effectiveness of proton pump inhibitors (PPIs), a common type of "acid" reflux medication.

If you are taking reflux medication, it is important to talk to your doctor before using peppermint.

17

SPICY FOODS

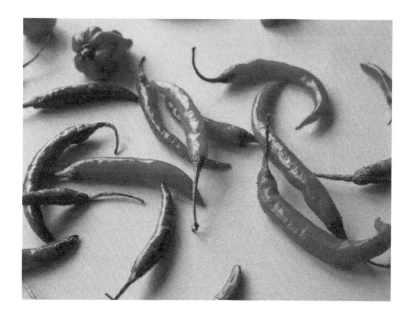

S picy foods are a common trigger for postnasal
drip. There are a few reasons why spicy foods can

make postnasal drip, throat clearing, mucus or phlegm in the throat, cough, voice crackling, sore throat, sense that the throat may close, feeling of a scratch or tickle in the throat, feeling of a lump in the throat, tight swallowing, food feeling like it is "going down the wrong pipe" and more worse:

- Spicy foods irritate the lining of the throat. The capsaicin in spicy foods can irritate the lining of the throat, making it more sensitive to stomach acid.
- Spicy foods slow down digestion. Spicy foods can slow down the emptying of the stomach. This means that pepsin, foodstuff, acid and bile stay in the stomach longer, increasing the risk of PND.
- Spicy foods relax the lower esophageal sphincter (LES). The LES is a muscle valve that separates the stomach from the throat. When the LES is relaxed, it is more likely to open and allow pepsin, foodstuff, acid and bile to back up into the throat.

Spicy foods make pepsin, foodstuff, acid and bile reflux worse in two ways. First, the capsaicin in many spicy foods can slow digestion. But before it even gets that far, it can irritate an already irritated throat on its way down.

HOW CAPSAICIN IRRITATES THE THROAT AND STOMACH

Capsaicin activates a receptor on the surface of cells called the transient receptor potential vanilloid 1 (TRPV1) receptor. TRPV1 receptors are found in a variety of tissues, including the throat, stomach, and throat. When capsaicin activates TRPV1 receptors, it causes the release of a neurotransmitter called calcitonin gene-related peptide (CGRP). CGRP is a vasodilator, which means that it widens blood vessels. This can lead to inflammation and pain.

In the throat, capsaicin can irritate the lining and cause postnasal drip, throat clearing, mucus or phlegm in the throat, cough, voice crackling, sore throat, sense that the throat may close, feeling of a scratch or tickle in the throat, feeling of a lump in the throat, tight swallowing, food feeling like it is "going down the wrong pipe" and more.. In the stomach, capsaicin can irritate the lining and cause ulcers. In the throat, capsaicin can irritate the lining and cause esophagitis – a significant swelling.

HOW CAPSAICIN SLOWS DOWN DIGESTION

Capsaicin can slow down digestion by relaxing the muscles of the stomach and intestines. This can give pepsin, foodstuff, acid and bile more time to back up into the throat.

How to reduce the risk of PND from spicy foods

If you have postnasal drip, throat clearing, mucus or phlegm in the throat, cough, voice crackling, sore throat, sense that the throat may close, feeling of a scratch or tickle in the throat, feeling of a lump in the throat, tight swallowing, food feeling like it is "going down the wrong pipe" and more, there are a few things you can do to reduce the risk of reflux from spicy foods:

- Avoid spicy foods altogether. This is the best way to prevent reflux from spicy foods.
- Limit your intake of spicy foods. If you can't resist spicy foods, try to limit your intake to small amounts.
- Choose less spicy foods. There are many different types of spicy foods. Some are spicier than others. Choose less spicy foods if you are prone to reflux.

- Eat spicy foods with other foods. Eating spicy foods with other foods can help to dilute the capsaicin and reduce its irritating effects.
- Avoid eating spicy foods before bed. Eating spicy foods before bed can increase the risk of reflux while you are sleeping.

It is important to note that not everyone who eats spicy foods will experience postnasal drip, throat clearing, mucus or phlegm in the throat, cough, voice crackling, sore throat, sense that the throat may close, feeling of a scratch or tickle in the throat, feeling of a lump in the throat, tight swallowing, food feeling like it is "going down the wrong pipe" and more. Some people are more sensitive to the capsaicin in spicy foods than others. If you are prone to PND, it is best to avoid spicy foods altogether or limit your intake to small amounts.

SECTION III

DOING

18

EAT SMALL MEALS

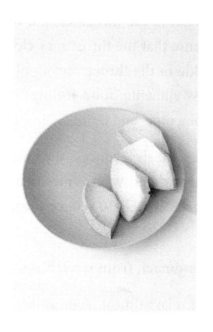

EATING SMALL MEALS CAN HELP THOSE WHO HAVE POSTNASAL DRIP IN A NUMBER OF WAYS.

Reduces the amount of chemicals in the throat

When you eat a large meal, your digestive system makes & secretes pepsin, bile, gastrin, acid and other chemicals to help break down the food. This excess of natural enzymes and chemicals irritate the lining of the throat and trigger postnasal drip, throat clearing, mucus or phlegm in the throat, cough, voice crackling, sore throat, sense that the throat may close, feeling of a scratch or tickle in the throat, feeling of a lump in the throat, tight swallowing, food feeling like it is "going down the wrong pipe" and more.

Eating smaller meals reduces the amount of acid, pepsin and other digestive enzymes that your stomach produces, which can help to reduce the risk of PND (& TSL).

Prevents the stomach from stretching

When you eat a large meal, your stomach stretches to accommodate the food. This stretching can relax the lower esophageal sphincter (LES), which is the muscle valve that separates the stomach from the throat. When the LES is relaxed, pepsin, foodstuff, acid and bile can back up into the throat, causing postnasal drip, throat clearing, mucus or phlegm in the throat, cough, voice crackling, sore throat, sense that the throat may close, feeling of a scratch or tickle in the throat, feeling of a lump in the throat, tight swallowing, food feeling like it is "going down the wrong pipe" and more.

Eating smaller meals helps to prevent the stomach from stretching and keeps the LES strong, which can help to reduce the risk of reflux.

Empties the stomach faster

Smaller meals empty the stomach faster than larger meals. This is because smaller meals are easier for the stomach to break down. When the stomach empties faster, there is less time for acid to build up and back up into the throat.

Reduces pressure in the abdomen

Eating a large meal can increase pressure in the abdomen. This increased pressure can push pepsin, foodstuff, acid and bile up into the throat, causing reflux. Eating smaller meals reduces pressure in the abdomen, which can help to reduce the risk of reflux.

As a side note, this seems to be the mechanism for obesity and pregnancy being causes of increased post-nasal drip, throat clearing, mucus or phlegm in the throat, cough, voice crackling, sore throat, sense that the throat may close, feeling of a scratch or tickle in the throat, feeling of a lump in the throat, tight swallowing, food feeling like it is "going down the wrong pipe" and more as well.

OTHER BENEFITS OF EATING SMALL MEALS

In addition to reducing the risk of reflux, eating small meals can also have a number of other health benefits, including:

- Weight loss or maintenance
- Improved blood sugar control
- Reduced risk of heart disease and stroke
- Increased energy levels
- Improved mood

HOW MANY SMALL MEALS SHOULD I EAT PER DAY?

There is no one-size-fits-all answer to this question, as the ideal number of small meals to eat per day will vary depending on the individual. However, most experts recommend eating four to six small meals per day. **If you would like to delve into this deeper, I recommend asking your HCW for a dietitian and/or nutrition consultation!**

Tips for eating small meals

- Eat three small meals and two or three snacks throughout the day.
- Make sure that your meals and snacks are balanced and contain a variety of foods from all food groups.
- Avoid eating large meals, especially before bed.
- Stop eating when you are about 80% full
- Eat slowly, SAVOR your food and chew your food thoroughly.
- Avoid drinking too much liquid with your meals, especially carbonated beverages and alcohol.

If you have reflux and you are starting to eat small meals, it is important to be patient. It may take some time for your body to adjust to the new eating schedule. However, **if you stick with it, you should start to see a reduction** in your postnasal drip, throat clearing, mucus or phlegm in the throat, cough, voice crackling, sore throat, sense that the throat may close, feeling of a scratch or tickle in the throat, feeling of a lump in the throat, tight swallowing, food feeling like it is "going down the wrong pipe" and more.

If you have any questions or concerns about eating small meals, please talk to your HCW or a registered dietitian.

19

GRAVITY

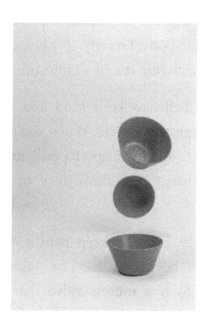

G ravity affects our digestion in a number of ways
and when you swallow, gravity helps to move

the food bolus (the ball of chewed food) down the throat and into the stomach. The esophagus is a muscular tube that connects the throat to the stomach. Gravity helps to open the lower esophageal sphincter (LES), which is a muscle valve that separates the esophagus from the stomach. The LES opens to allow the food bolus to pass into the stomach, and then closes to prevent pepsin, foodstuff, acid and bile from backing up into the throat.

Gravity helps to mix food with gastric juices in the stomach. Gastric juices are acids and enzymes that help to break down food into smaller pieces that can be absorbed by the body. Gravity also helps to move food from the stomach into the small intestine.

First, gravity helps to keep food and liquid moving through the digestive system. When you are standing or sitting upright, gravity helps to pull food and liquid down your throat and through your stomach and intestines.

Second, gravity helps to keep pepsin, foodstuff, acid and bile in the stomach. The lower esophageal sphincter (LES) is a muscle valve that separates the stomach from the throat. Gravity helps to keep the LES closed, which prevents pepsin, foodstuff, acid and bile from backing up into the throat.

Third, gravity helps to keep the stomach from emptying too quickly. When you are standing or sitting upright, gravity helps to keep food in the stomach longer. This allows the stomach to have more time to digest the food.

HOW GRAVITY CAN CONTRIBUTE TO POSTNASAL DRIP

Gravity can contribute to reflux in a number of ways. First, when you are lying down, gravity is no longer pulling food and liquid down your digestive system. This can cause pepsin, foodstuff, acid and bile to back up into your throat, which can lead to reflux.

Second, when you are lying down, the LES is under less pressure from gravity. This can make it more likely for the LES to relax and allow pepsin, foodstuff, acid and bile to back up into the throat.

Third, when you are lying down, the stomach can empty more quickly. This can lead to a sudden influx of pepsin, foodstuff, acid and bile into the throat, which can cause postnasal drip, throat clearing, mucus or phlegm in the throat, cough, voice crackling, sore throat, sense that the throat may close, feeling of a scratch or tickle in the throat, feeling of a lump in the throat, tight swallowing, food feeling like it is "going down the wrong pipe" and more.

WHY ELEVATING THE HEAD OF THE BED HELPS THOSE WHO HAVE REFLUX

Elevating the head of the bed can help to prevent reflux in a number of ways.

First, elevating the head of the bed helps to keep food and liquid moving down your digestive system. This is because gravity is pulling food and liquid down your throat and through your stomach and intestines.

Second, elevating the head of the bed helps to keep the LES closed. This is because gravity is putting pressure on the LES.

Third, elevating the head of the bed helps to keep the stomach from emptying too quickly. This is because gravity is keeping food in the stomach longer.

HOW TO ELEVATE THE HEAD OF THE BED

There are a number of ways to elevate the head of the bed. One way is to place a [bed] wedge under the mattress. Another way is to use a **bed rest**. You can also place a few pillows under your head and shoulders. However, there are two issues with these three options.

First, I have seen a patient who had osteoporosis obtain a compression fracture of her spine that she was convinced had to do with the bed wedge. And second, if the entire torso is not elevated on an angle, then it is unlikely to be effective.

If you have postnasal drip, throat clearing, mucus or phlegm in the throat, cough, voice crackling, sore throat, sense that the throat may close, feeling of a scratch or tickle in the throat, feeling of a lump in the throat, tight swallowing, food feeling like it is "going down the wrong pipe" and more, it can be important to elevate the head of your bed by at least 6 inches. This will help to prevent pepsin, foodstuff, acid and bile from backing up into your throat.

The BEST way is to either have a mattress that is on an angle from head to toe (an adjustable bed) or to use something dense like a cinder block placed under each head poster of the bed frame to get that nice angle of the torso so that gravity can work through the night.

There is some risk with this best option, however. First, you might need help to get the blocks in because they can be heavy; next, you might need to cover them for aesthetics and/or for the sake of not leaving marks in your floor, and lastly, be sure to test out the bed before lying your whole body on it to be sure it is safe and sturdy.

20

WATER AT NIGHT

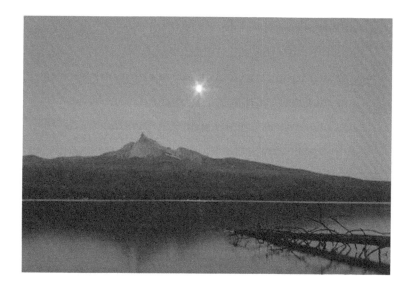

Eating or drinking anything but water for hours before bedtime can trigger postnasal drip, throat clearing, mucus or phlegm in the throat, cough, voice crackling, sore throat, sense that the throat may close, feeling of a scratch or tickle in the throat, feeling of a lump in the throat, tight swallowing, food feeling like it is "going down the wrong pipe" and more in a number of ways:

- Certain food and drinks (see section one above) can relax the lower esophageal sphincter (LES): The LES is a muscle valve that separates the stomach from the throat. When the LES is relaxed, pepsin, foodstuff, acid and bile can back up into the throat, causing reflux. Food and drinks, especially those that are high in fat, acid, or caffeine, can relax the LES.
- Certain food and drinks (see section one above) can increase stomach acid production: When you eat or drink, your stomach produces acid to help break down the food. This increased acid production can lead to PND.
- Certain food and drinks (see section one above) can delay gastric emptying: Gastric emptying is the process of food moving from the stomach into the small intestine. When gastric emptying is delayed, food stays in the stomach for a longer period of time. The longer food stays in the stomach, the more time it has to produce pepsin, acid and bile.

Avoiding food and drinks for hours before bedtime can help to reduce the risk of reflux by:

- Keeping the LES closed: When you are not eating or drinking, your stomach is empty and the LES is more likely to stay closed. This helps to prevent stomach pepsin, foodstuff, acid and bile from backing up into the throat.
- Reducing stomach acid production: When you are not eating or drinking, your stomach is not producing acid. This helps to reduce the amount of acid in your stomach and reduce the risk of reflux.
- Promoting gastric emptying: When you are not eating or drinking, your stomach can empty more quickly. This helps to reduce the amount of time that food stays in your stomach and reduce the risk of PND.

HOW LONG SHOULD YOU AVOID EATING AND DRINKING BEFORE BED IF YOU HAVE REFLUX?

It is recommended that you avoid eating and drinking anything but water for at least 3-4 hours before bedtime if you have reflux. This will give your stomach time to empty and reduce the risk of reflux.

If you find that you are still experiencing postnasal drip, throat clearing, mucus or phlegm in the throat, cough, voice crackling, sore throat, sense that the throat may close, feeling of a scratch or tickle in the throat, feeling of a lump in the throat, tight swallowing, food feeling like it is "going down the wrong pipe" and more after avoiding food and drinks for 3-4 hours before bedtime, you may need to extend the amount of time that you avoid eating and drinking before bed.

Here are some tips for avoiding food and drinks before bed if you have PND:

- Eat your last meal of the day at least 3-4 hours before bedtime.
- Avoid snacks and late-night meals.
- Avoid drinking alcohol, caffeine, and carbonated beverages before bed.
- Drink plenty of water throughout the day, but avoid drinking too much water before bed.

If you are thirsty before bed, **only drink water**. You should avoid other drinks, such as:

- Coffee
- Tea
- Soda
- Alcohol

- Juice
- Fatty milk
- Chocolate milk

These drinks can all relax the LES and increase the risk of postnasal drip & TSL.

If you have to have a specific beverage (for example, a diabetic who need a sugar drink), then please discuss this with your nurse, HCW, dietitian or nutritionist!

21

ABDOMINAL PRESSURE

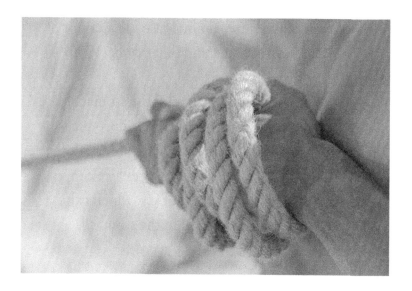

Avoiding body positions and activities that increase abdominal ("belly") pressure can help to reduce the risk of postnasal drip in a number of ways:

- Reduces pressure on the lower esophageal sphincter (LES): The LES is a muscle valve that separates the stomach from the throat. When the LES is relaxed, pepsin, foodstuff, acid and bile can back up into the esophagus. Increased abdominal pressure can relax the LES and make it more likely for pepsin, foodstuff, acid and bile to back up.

- Reduces the amount of pepsin, foodstuff, acid and bile that backs up into the throat: When the LES is relaxed, pepsin, foodstuff, acid and bile can back up into the throat. Increased abdominal pressure can increase the amount of pepsin, foodstuff, acid and bile that backs up into the throat.

- Reduces the amount of food in the stomach: When you eat a meal, your stomach produces pepsin, acid and moves bile to help break down the food. Increased abdominal pressure can empty the stomach more quickly, which can reduce the amount of food in the stomach.

SPECIFIC BODY POSITIONS AND ACTIVITIES TO AVOID

Some specific body positions and activities to avoid to reduce the risk of postnasal drip include:

- Bending over: Bending over increases abdominal pressure, which can relax the LES and increase the amount of pepsin, foodstuff, acid and bile that backs up into the throat.
- Certain types of Exercising: Exercise, especially strenuous exercise, can increase abdominal pressure. If you have reflux, it is important to choose low-impact exercises and avoid exercises that put a lot of strain on your abdomen.
- Singing: Singing can increase abdominal pressure, which can relax the LES and increase the amount of pepsin, foodstuff, acid and bile that backs up into the throat.
- Sitting: Sitting can increase abdominal pressure, especially if you have a lot of weight in your abdomen. If you sit for long periods of time, try to get up and move around every 20-30 minutes.
- Wearing a belt, corset, or tight underwear: Wearing a belt, corset, or tight underwear can

increase abdominal pressure. If you have reflux, try to wear loose-fitting clothing.

BODY POSITIONS AND ACTIVITIES THAT INCREASE ABDOMINAL PRESSURE

Some body positions and activities that increase abdominal pressure include:

- Bending over
- Exercising
- Lifting heavy objects
- Straining to have a bowel movement
- Wearing tight clothing, such as belts, corsets, and tight underwear
- Pregnancy
- Being overweight

How to reduce the risk of PND by avoiding body positions and activities that increase abdominal pressure

If you have postnasal drip, throat clearing, mucus or phlegm in the throat, cough, voice crackling, sore throat, sense that the throat may close, feeling of a scratch or tickle in the throat, feeling of a lump in the throat, tight swallowing, food feeling like it is "going down the wrong pipe" and more, it is important to avoid body positions and activities that increase abdominal pressure. This includes:

- Bending over
- Exercising too intensely
- Lifting heavy objects
- Straining to have a bowel movement
- Wearing tight clothing, such as belts, corsets, and tight underwear

Avoiding body positions and activities that increase abdominal pressure can help to reduce the risk of reflux by reducing pressure on the LES, reducing the amount of pepsin, foodstuff, acid and bile that backs up into the throat, and reducing the amount of food in the stomach.

Other tips for reducing the risk of postnasal drip, throat clearing, mucus or phlegm in the throat, cough, voice crackling, sore throat, sense that the throat may close, feeling of a scratch or tickle in the throat, feeling of a lump in the throat, tight swallowing, food feeling like it is "going down the wrong pipe" and more include eating small, frequent meals, avoiding eating before bed, elevating the head of your bed, and avoiding foods and drinks that trigger reflux.

22

WHY EXERCISE AND WEIGHT LOSS HELP

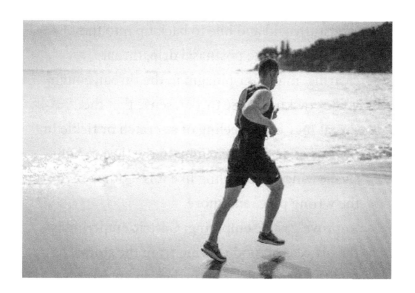

E xercise and weight loss can help to reduce the risk of postnasal drip in a number of ways:

- Reduce pressure on the LES: The lower esophageal sphincter (LES) is a muscle valve that separates the stomach from the throat. When you are overweight or obese, the increased pressure in your abdomen can push the LES open and allow pepsin, foodstuff, acid and bile to back up into the throat. Exercise and weight loss can help to reduce pressure on the LES and keep it closed.
- Strengthen the esophageal muscles: Exercise can help to strengthen the esophageal muscles, which can make it more difficult for pepsin, foodstuff, acid and bile to back up into the throat and create postnasal drip, throat clearing, mucus or phlegm in the throat, cough, voice crackling, sore throat, sense that the throat may close, feeling of a scratch or tickle in the throat, feeling of a lump in the throat, tight swallowing, food feeling like it is "going down the wrong pipe" and more.
- Improve gastric emptying: Gastric emptying is the process of food moving from the stomach into the small intestine further down. Exercise can help to improve gastric emptying, which can reduce the amount of time that pepsin, foodstuff, acid and bile has to back up into the throat.

- Reduce inflammation: Exercise can help to reduce inflammation in the throat, which can make it less sensitive to pepsin, foodstuff, acid and bile.

In addition to helping to reduce the risk of postnasal drip and TSL, exercise and weight loss can also improve other digestive symptoms, such as bloating, gas, and indigestion.

WHAT TYPE OF EXERCISE IS BEST FOR PEOPLE WITH PND?

Moderate-intensity exercise is best for people with postnasal drip and such TSL symptoms. This type of exercise can help to improve gastric emptying and reduce pressure on the LES without causing too much abdominal pressure.

Good examples of moderate-intensity exercise for people with reflux include:

- Walking
- Biking
- Swimming
- Tai Chi
- Pilates

Consider avoiding exercises that increase abdominal pressure, such as:

- Weightlifting
- Crunches
- Sit-ups
- Running

HOW MUCH EXERCISE SHOULD PEOPLE WITH REFLUX DO?

The Centers for Disease Control and Prevention (CDC) recommends that adults get at least 150 minutes of moderate-intensity aerobic activity or 75 minutes of vigorous-intensity aerobic activity each week.

If you are new to exercise, start slowly and gradually increase the amount of time you exercise each week. It is also important to listen to your body and rest when you need to.

HOW TO START AN EXERCISE PROGRAM IF YOU HAVE PND

If you have postnasal drip, throat clearing, mucus or phlegm in the throat, cough, voice crackling, sore throat, sense that the throat may close, feeling of a scratch or tickle in the throat, feeling of a lump in the throat, tight swallowing, food feeling like it is "going down the wrong pipe" and more and are new to exercise, it is important to start slowly and gradually increase the intensity and duration of your workouts. It is also important to listen to your body and stop exercising if you experience any of the PND symptoms.

Here are some tips for starting an exercise program if you have PND:

- Start with low-impact exercises.
- Gradually increase the intensity and duration of your workouts.
- Listen to your body and stop exercising if you experience any throat symptoms.
- Avoid exercises that increase abdominal pressure.
- Eat a healthy diet (see section 1 of this book) and maintain a healthy weight.
- Avoid eating before exercising.
- Drink plenty of water before, during, and after exercising.

HOW MUCH WEIGHT LOSS IS NEEDED TO IMPROVE POSTNASAL DRIP & TSL SYMPTOMS?

Even a small amount of weight loss can improve post-nasal drip, throat clearing, mucus or phlegm in the throat, cough, voice crackling, sore throat, sense that the throat may close, feeling of a scratch or tickle in the throat, feeling of a lump in the throat, tight swallowing, food feeling like it is "going down the wrong pipe" and more symptoms. In one study, people who lost just 5-10% of their body weight experienced a significant reduction in reflux symptoms.

If you are overweight or obese, talk to your doctor about a safe and effective way to lose weight.

Exercise and weight loss can help to reduce the risk of reflux and improve other digestive symptoms. If you have reflux, talk to your doctor about a safe and effective exercise and weight loss plan.

23

FASTING AND HORMESIS

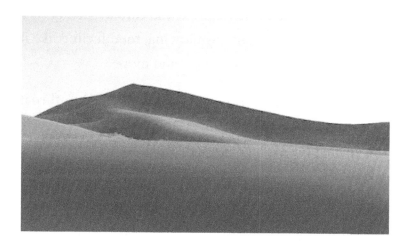

FASTING

F asting is the voluntary abstinence from food and drink for a period of time. It has been practiced for centuries for both religious and health reasons. In recent years, there has been growing interest in the health benefits of fasting.

One of the ways that fasting can help those with post-nasal drip is by reducing the amount of stomach acid that is produced. When you eat, your stomach produces acid to help break down the food. However, too much stomach acid can back up into the throat, causing PND. Fasting can help to reduce stomach acid production, which can lead to a decrease in postnasal drip, throat clearing, mucus or phlegm in the throat, cough, voice crackling, sore throat, sense that the throat may close, feeling of a scratch or tickle in the throat, feeling of a lump in the throat, tight swallowing, food feeling like it is "going down the wrong pipe" and more.

Another way that fasting can help with PND & throat symptoms is by promoting weight loss. We discussed this in chapter 21.

Fasting also gives the throat a chance to heal. If your throat is irritated from mucus, fasting can give it a chance to heal. This is because fasting reduces the amount of pepsin, foodstuff, acid and bile that comes into contact with the lining of the throat.

HORMESIS

Hormesis is a biological phenomenon in which exposure to a low "dose" of a stressor can have a beneficial effect. For example, exercise is a form of hormesis, as it puts stress on the body but leads to improved health outcomes in the long term.

One way that hormesis can help with PND is by strengthening the lower esophageal sphincter (LES). The LES is a muscle valve that separates the stomach from the throat. When the LES is weak, it is more likely to open and allow pepsin, foodstuff, acid and bile to back up into the throat. Hormesis can help to strengthen the LES and reduce the risk of postnasal drip, throat clearing, mucus or phlegm in the throat, cough, voice crackling, sore throat, sense that the throat may close, feeling of a scratch or tickle in the throat, feeling of a lump in the throat, tight swallowing, food feeling like it is "going down the wrong pipe" and more.

Another way that hormesis can help with postnasal drip, throat clearing, mucus or phlegm in the throat, cough, voice crackling, sore throat, sense that the throat may close, feeling of a scratch or tickle in the throat, feeling of a lump in the throat, tight swallowing, food feeling like it is "going down the wrong pipe" and more is by **reducing inflammation**. Inflammation is a process that occurs in the body in response to injury or infection.

However, chronic inflammation can contribute to a number of health problems, including postnasal drip and TSL. Hormesis can help to reduce inflammation throughout the body, and therefore can be used as an indirect treatment for it.

HOW TO FAST AND PRACTICE HORMESIS FOR PND

There are a number of different ways to fast. One popular method is intermittent fasting, which involves alternating between periods of eating and fasting. Another popular method is extended fasting, which involves fasting for 24 hours or more.

If you are new to fasting, it is important to start slowly and gradually increase the duration of your fasts. It is also important to listen to your body and stop fasting if you experience any negative side effects.

Here are some tips for fasting safely:

- Start with short fasts, such as a 12-hour fast overnight.

- Gradually increase the duration of your fasts as you become more comfortable.
- Drink plenty of water and other unsweetened beverages during your fast.
- Listen to your body and stop fasting if you experience any negative side effects.

To practice hormesis for PND, you can engage in low-intensity exercise on a regular basis. You can also expose yourself to other mild stressors, such as cold exposure or sauna bathing.

CONCLUSION

Fasting and hormesis are two promising approaches to managing postnasal drip, throat clearing, mucus or phlegm in the throat, cough, voice crackling, sore throat, sense that the throat may close, feeling of a scratch or tickle in the throat, feeling of a lump in the throat, tight swallowing, food feeling like it is "going down the wrong pipe" and more. Fasting can help to reduce stomach acid production, promote weight loss, and strengthen the LES. Hormesis can help to reduce inflammation and strengthen the LES.

If you are considering trying fasting or hormesis, it is important to talk to your HCW first.

24

SLEEP QUALITY AND THE TREATMENT OF SLEEP APNEA

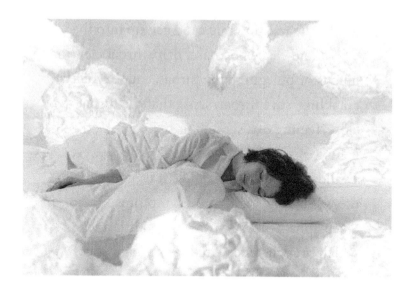

HOW SLEEP QUALITY AND SLEEP APNEA CAN AFFECT POSTNASAL DRIP

Sleep quality and sleep apnea can affect PND in a number of ways.

- Sleep quality: When you don't get enough sleep, your body produces more of the stress hormone cortisol. Cortisol can relax the lower esophageal sphincter (LES), which is the muscle valve that separates the stomach from the throat. When the LES is relaxed, pepsin, foodstuff, acid and bile can back up into the throat and cause postnasal drip, throat clearing, mucus or phlegm in the throat, cough, voice crackling, sore throat, sense that the throat may close, feeling of a scratch or tickle in the throat, feeling of a lump in the throat, tight swallowing, food feeling like it is "going down the wrong pipe" and more symptoms.
- Sleep apnea: Sleep apnea is a condition in which breathing repeatedly stops and starts during sleep. Sleep apnea can increase the risk of postnasal drip, throat clearing, mucus or phlegm in the throat, cough, voice crackling, sore throat, sense that the throat may close, feeling of a scratch or tickle in the throat,

feeling of a lump in the throat, tight swallowing, food feeling like it is "going down the wrong pipe" and more by:

- Reducing the production of saliva, which helps to neutralize stomach contents.
- Increasing the amount of negative pressure in the chest, which can push pepsin, foodstuff, acid and bile up into the throat.
- Disrupting sleep, which can lead to increased cortisol production and a relaxed LES.

HOW ADEQUATE SLEEP QUALITY AND THE TREATMENT OF SLEEP APNEA WITH POSITIVE PRESSURE CAN HELP PND

Adequate sleep quality and the treatment of sleep apnea with positive pressure can help postnasal drip, throat clearing, mucus or phlegm in the throat, cough, voice crackling, sore throat, sense that the throat may close, feeling of a scratch or tickle in the throat, feeling of a lump in the throat, tight swallowing, food feeling like it is "going down the wrong pipe" and more in a number of ways:

- Reduces stomach acid production. When you don't get enough sleep, your body produces more of the stress hormone cortisol. Cortisol can increase stomach acid production. Getting enough sleep can help to reduce cortisol levels and stomach acid production.

- Improves digestion. Sleep is important for digestion. When you don't get enough sleep, your digestive system doesn't work as well. This can lead to a number of problems, including postnasal drip and throat symptoms. Getting enough sleep can help to improve digestion and reduce the risk of PND.

- Strengthens the lower esophageal sphincter (LES). The LES is the muscle valve that separates the stomach from the throat. When the LES is weak, it is more likely to open and allow pepsin, foodstuff, acid and bile to back up into the throat. Adequate sleep and the treatment of sleep apnea with positive pressure can help to strengthen the LES and reduce the risk of postnasal drip and throat symptoms.

Adequate sleep quality and the treatment of sleep apnea with positive pressure can help PND in a number of ways:

- Adequate sleep quality: When you get enough sleep, your body produces less cortisol and more saliva. This helps to strengthen the LES and reduce the risk of postnasal drip, throat clearing, mucus or phlegm in the throat, cough, voice crackling, sore throat, sense that the throat may close, feeling of a scratch or tickle in the throat, feeling of a lump in the throat, tight swallowing, food feeling like it is "going down the wrong pipe" and more.

- Treatment of sleep apnea with positive pressure: Positive pressure therapy is the most effective treatment for sleep apnea. Positive pressure therapy works by using a mask to deliver pressurized air to the throat during sleep. This helps to keep the airway open and prevent breathing from stopping and starting. Treating sleep apnea with positive pressure can help to reduce the risk of PND by:
- Increasing the production of saliva.
- Reducing the amount of negative pressure in the chest.
- Improving sleep quality.

HOW TO IMPROVE SLEEP QUALITY

There are a number of things you can do to improve your sleep quality:

- Stick to a regular sleep schedule. Go to bed and wake up at the same time each day, even on weekends.
- Create a relaxing bedtime routine. This could include taking a warm bath, reading a book, or listening to calming music.
- Make sure your bedroom is dark, quiet, and cool.
- Avoid caffeine and alcohol before bed (see chapters 9 and 10)
- Get regular exercise, but avoid exercising too close to bedtime.

HOW TO TREAT SLEEP APNEA WITH POSITIVE PRESSURE

If you have sleep apnea, you will need to see a doctor to get a diagnosis and treatment plan. The most effective treatment for sleep apnea is positive pressure therapy. Positive pressure therapy works by using a mask to deliver pressurized air to the throat during sleep. This helps to keep the airway open and prevent breathing from stopping and starting.

There is also a theoretical treatment element here: while the positive airway pressure is designed to keep the airway open, it can also "give pressure" to the upper throat to prevent pepsin, foodstuff, acid and bile from entering the throat and leading to postnasal drip, throat clearing, mucus or phlegm in the throat, cough, voice crackling, sore throat, sense that the throat may close, feeling of a scratch or tickle in the throat, feeling of a lump in the throat, tight swallowing, food feeling like it is "going down the wrong pipe" and more.

Also, in the "art of medicine" it is common to think of reflux and sleep apnea as synergistic or symbiotic diseases:

If you have PND & reflux, then sleep apnea symptoms are usually worse and conversely, if you have sleep apnea, then often postnasal drip and TSL are worse.

Your HCW will work with you to determine which type of positive pressure therapy is right for you. At this time, it is unclear if oral appliances or hypoglossal nerve surgery has an effect on throat symptoms.

Adequate sleep quality and the treatment of sleep apnea with positive pressure can help to reduce the risk of postnasal drip, throat clearing, mucus or phlegm in the throat, cough, voice crackling, sore throat, sense that the throat may close, feeling of a scratch or tickle in the throat, feeling of a lump in the throat, tight swallowing, food feeling like it is "going down the wrong pipe" and more. If you have PND, talk to your doctor about how to improve your sleep quality and whether sleep testing and/or positive pressure therapy is right for you.

SECTION IV

MEDICINE

25

WATER AND ALKALINE WATER

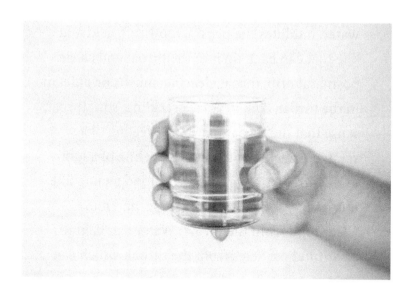

B oth water and alkaline water may help those who have postnasal drip, but in different ways.

WATER

Water is essential for good health and can help with a variety of health problems, including postnasal drip, throat clearing, mucus or phlegm in the throat, cough, voice crackling, sore throat, sense that the throat may close, feeling of a scratch or tickle in the throat, feeling of a lump in the throat, tight swallowing, food feeling like it is "going down the wrong pipe" and more. Water helps to:

- Dilute stomach contents: When you drink water, it dilutes the pepsin, foodstuff, acid and bile that can back up into the throat and cause postnasal drip, throat clearing, mucus or phlegm in the throat, cough, voice crackling, sore throat, sense that the throat may close, feeling of a scratch or tickle in the throat, feeling of a lump in the throat, tight swallowing, food feeling like it is "going down the wrong pipe" and more.
- Clear food from the throat: Water can help to clear food particles from the throat, which can reduce irritation and inflammation.
- Promote digestion: Water helps to promote digestion by moving food through the digestive system more efficiently.

- Flush pepsin, foodstuff, acid and bile out of the throat.
- Promote digestion.
- Keep the throat moist and reduce irritation.
- Reduce the amount of time pepsin, foodstuff, acid and bile is in contact with the lining of the throat: The longer pepsin, foodstuff, acid and bile is in contact with the lining of the throat, the more likely they are to cause irritation. Drinking water can help to reduce the amount of time these chemicals are in contact with the lining of the throat.

ALKALINE WATER

Alkaline water has a higher pH level than regular water. pH is a measure of how acidic or alkaline a substance is. A pH of 7 is neutral, a pH below 7 is acidic, and a pH above 7 is alkaline.

Some people believe that alkaline water can help to neutralize stomach acid and reduce postnasal drip, throat clearing, mucus or phlegm in the throat, cough, voice crackling, sore throat, sense that the throat may close, feeling of a scratch or tickle in the throat, feeling of a lump in the throat, tight swallowing, food feeling like it is "going down the wrong pipe" and more.

However, there is limited scientific evidence to support this claim.

One thing is for sure – the use of alkaline water is to neutralize pepsin, foodstuff, acid and bile. *It does not and will not change the pH of blood which some have claimed.*

HOW MUCH WATER SHOULD I DRINK TO HELP WITH PND?

It is important to drink plenty of fluids throughout the day to help with postnasal drip and TSL. If you are drinking alkaline water, there is no specific recommendation for how much to drink. However, it is important to start slowly and gradually increase your intake to avoid any side effects.

How to choose alkaline water

If you choose to drink alkaline water, there are a few things to keep in mind:

- Choose alkaline water with a pH level of 8.0-9.0: This is the pH range that is most likely to be beneficial for PND.
- Avoid alkaline water with added ingredients: Some alkaline water products contain added ingredients, such as minerals or antioxidants.

There is no evidence that these ingredients are beneficial for reflux.

- Talk to your doctor: Before drinking alkaline water, talk to your doctor to make sure it is safe for you.

Both water and alkaline water may help those who have postnasal drip, throat clearing, mucus or phlegm in the throat, cough, voice crackling, sore throat, sense that the throat may close, feeling of a scratch or tickle in the throat, feeling of a lump in the throat, tight swallowing, food feeling like it is "going down the wrong pipe" and more. Water helps to dilute stomach acid, clear food from the throat, and promote digestion. Alkaline water may help to neutralize stomach acid and reduce PND symptoms.

If you choose to drink alkaline water, start slowly and gradually increase your intake to avoid any side effects. Talk to your HCW before drinking alkaline water to make sure it is safe for you.

26

SUGAR-FREE GUM AND MANUKA HONEY LOZENGES

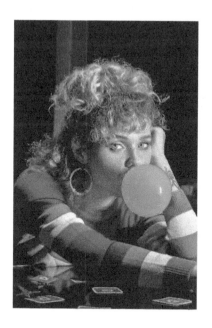

CHEWING SUGAR-FREE GUM (SFG)

C hewing sugar-free gum can help to relieve PND symptoms in a number of ways:

- Increases saliva production: Saliva is a natural antacid that can help to neutralize pepsin, foodstuff, acid and bile and reduce the amount of these chemicals that back up into the throat. Chewing sugar-free gum increases saliva production, which can help to reduce postnasal drip, throat clearing, mucus or phlegm in the throat, cough, voice crackling, sore throat, sense that the throat may close, feeling of a scratch or tickle in the throat, feeling of a lump in the throat, tight swallowing, food feeling like it is "going down the wrong pipe" and more (TSL).

- Strengthens the lower esophageal sphincter (LES): The LES is the muscle valve that separates the stomach from the throat. When the LES is weak, it is more likely to open and allow pepsin, foodstuff, acid and bile to back up into the throat. Chewing sugar-free gum can help to strengthen the LES and reduce the risk of postnasal drip and TSL.

- Empties the stomach faster: Chewing sugar-free gum can help to empty the stomach faster, which reduces the amount of time that pepsin, foodstuff, acid and bile is in contact with the lining of the throat. This can help to reduce postnasal drip and TSL.
- The main cavity-causing bacteria in the mouth is called *Streptococcus Mutans*. When we consume sugary foods and drinks, more of this type of bacteria gets converted into acids that attack our teeth. Consumption of **xylitol** in many SFG helps to slow down the production of *Streptococcus Mutans*, thereby reducing acid production. Xylitol also helps to neutralize the pH of the saliva, reducing the acidity. The amount of acid-producing bacteria in our mouths can reduce as much as 90% after the use of a xylitol-containing product.

MANUKA HONEY LOZENGES

Manuka honey is a type of honey that is produced by bees in New Zealand. Manuka honey has antimicrobial and anti-inflammatory properties, which may be helpful for people with postnasal drip, throat clearing, mucus or phlegm in the throat, cough, voice crackling, sore throat, sense that the throat may close, feeling of a scratch or tickle in the throat, feeling of a lump in the throat, tight swallowing, food feeling like it is "going down the wrong pipe" and more.

Manuka honey lozenges can help to relieve PND symptoms in a number of ways:

- Coats & soothes the lining of the throat: Manuka honey can coat the lining of the throat and protect it from irritation from pepsin, foodstuff, acid and bile.
- Creates a barrier on the lining of the throat: Manuka honey can create a thin barrier on the lining of the throat. This barrier can help to protect the lining of the throat from pepsin, foodstuff, acid and bile.
- Reduces inflammation: Manuka honey has anti-inflammatory properties, which can help to reduce inflammation in the throat caused by pepsin, foodstuff, acid and bile.
- Kills bacteria: Manuka honey has antimicrobial properties, which can help to kill harmful bacteria in the throat. This may be especially helpful for people with postnasal drip and other throat symptoms.

HOW TO USE CHEWING SUGAR-FREE GUM AND MANUKA HONEY LOZENGES FOR PND

If you have PND & TSL, you can try chewing sugar-free gum and sucking on manuka honey lozenges to relieve your symptoms.

Here are some tips:

- Chew sugar-free gum for at least 30 minutes after meals.
- Suck on manuka honey lozenges throughout the day, especially after meals and before bed.
- Choose sugar-free gum and manuka honey lozenges that contain at least 10% manuka honey.

Chewing sugar-free gum and using manuka honey lozenges can both help to relieve postnasal drip and throat symptoms. Sugar-free gum can help to increase saliva production, strengthen the LES, and reduce the amount of time pepsin, foodstuff, acid and bile is in contact with the lining of the throat. Manuka honey can help to soothe the lining of the throat, neutralize stomach acid, and create a barrier on the lining of the throat.

However, it is important to note that more research is needed to confirm these benefits.

27

GAVISCON ADVANCE ANISEED

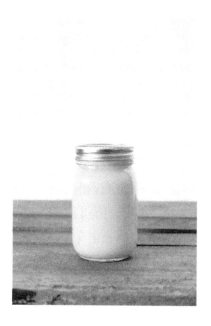

G aviscon Advance Aniseed is a liquid or tablet over-the-counter (OTC) medicine that is used to treat postnasal drip, throat clearing, mucus or phlegm in the throat, cough, voice crackling, sore throat, sense that the throat may close, feeling of a scratch or tickle in the throat, feeling of a lump in the throat, tight swallowing, food feeling like it is "going down the wrong pipe" and more. It works by forming a protective layer over the stomach contents, which prevents pepsin, foodstuff, acid and bile from backing up into the throat.

Gaviscon Advance Aniseed contains two active ingredients: sodium alginate and potassium bicarbonate.

- Sodium alginate is a natural substance that is derived from seaweed. It reacts with stomach acid to form a thick gel-like substance. This gel floats on top of the stomach contents and prevents pepsin, foodstuff, acid and bile from backing up into the throat.
- Potassium bicarbonate is an antacid that neutralizes stomach acid. This can help to relieve postnasal drip and TSL.

Gaviscon Advance Aniseed is available in two forms: a liquid and a tablet. The liquid form is more effective than the tablet form, but it can have a chalky taste. The tablet form is less effective than the liquid form, but it is easier to take and has a more pleasant taste.

HOW TO USE GAVISCON ADVANCE ANISEED FOR PND

Like every medicine, including OTC medicines, it is important to speak with your pharmacist to be sure this is right for you.

To use Gaviscon Advance Aniseed for postnasal drip, throat clearing, mucus or phlegm in the throat, cough, voice crackling, sore throat, sense that the throat may close, feeling of a scratch or tickle in the throat, feeling of a lump in the throat, tight swallowing, food feeling like it is "going down the wrong pipe" and more, take one or two doses of the liquid or two to four tablets after meals and before bed. You can also take Gaviscon Advance Aniseed between meals if you are experiencing PND symptoms. This is not a prescription medicine. It is typically taken after meals and before bed. The recommended dose is 10-20 ml for adults and children over 12 years old. Children under 12 years old should talk to their doctor about the appropriate dose.

To take liquid Gaviscon Advance Aniseed, shake the bottle well and measure out the recommended dose. Pour the medication into a spoon and drink it slowly. You can also take Gaviscon Advance Aniseed directly from the bottle.

SIDE EFFECTS OF GAVISCON ADVANCE ANISEED

Gaviscon Advance Aniseed is generally safe and well-tolerated. However, it can cause some side effects, such as:

- Constipation
- Diarrhea
- Stomach cramps
- Bloating
- Gas
- Chalky taste (liquid form only)

If you experience any side effects from Gaviscon Advance Aniseed, talk to your HCW.

BENEFITS OF USING GAVISCON ADVANCE ANISEED FOR PND

Gaviscon Advance Aniseed has a number of benefits for people with PND, including:

- It is a fast-acting medication. Relief from PND symptoms typically begins within minutes of taking Gaviscon Advance Aniseed.

- It is a long-lasting medication. Relief from PND symptoms can last for up to four hours after taking Gaviscon Advance Aniseed.
- It is a safe and effective medication for most people. Gaviscon Advance Aniseed is generally well-tolerated and has few side effects.
- It is a convenient medication. Gaviscon Advance Aniseed is available in a liquid form that is easy to take.

Additional information

- Gaviscon Advance Aniseed is available over-the-counter in most pharmacies. It is important to read the label carefully and follow the instructions before using it.
- If you have any questions or concerns about using Gaviscon Advance Aniseed, talk to your doctor or pharmacist.

Gaviscon Advance Aniseed appears to be an effective treatment for postnasal drip and more throat symptoms. It works by forming a protective layer over the stomach contents and neutralizing stomach acid specifically. Gaviscon Advance Aniseed is generally safe and well-tolerated, but it can cause some side effects such as constipation, diarrhea, and stomach cramps. Talk to your HCW before using this.

And remember, you can obtain the CTL by stopping certain things (see section I) and doing others (section II). Your best next step after full medical evaluation by your HCW is in sections I and II, not going right for this "medicine"!

28

MISCELLANEOUS REMEDIES

HERBS

Ginger

Ginger is one of the best digestive aids because of its medicinal properties. It's alkaline in nature and anti-inflammatory, which eases irritation in the digestive tract. Try sipping ginger tea when you feel heartburn coming on.

Ginger has medicinal properties and anti-inflammatory properties that make it one of the best digestive aids. It's alkaline, which means that it falls on the opposite side of the pH scale than acidic foods. Ginger is one of the foods that can neutralize stomach acid immediately.

The low level of pH eases irritation in the gastrointestinal tract. Ginger has been used throughout history for digestive issues. Ginger can be added to smoothies, soups, stir fry, or other dishes, or steeped as a tea.

Parsley

That sprig of parsley on your plate isn't just for decoration. Parsley has been a traditional treatment for upset stomach for hundreds of years.

Aloe vera

This is another old treatment for throat symptoms: one can buy aloe vera as a plant or as a supplement -- in capsules, juices, and other forms. It works as a thickener in recipes. Just make sure it's free of *anthraquinones* (primarily the compound aloin), which can be irritating to the digestive system.

NB:

There are many videos on social media and streaming about "this and that" remedy. More work is being done to find such herbs or "natural remedies", and future editions of this book will look into those. Suffice it to say that many of these (e.g. iberis, caraway, chamomile, mushroom cap, lion's mane, deglycyrrhizinated licorice root, etc.) are not ready for inclusion in this list.

FOODS

Good news: There are plenty of foods you can eat to help prevent postnasal drip and more throat symptoms (TSL). Stock your kitchen with foods from these three categories:

High-fiber foods

Fibrous foods make you feel full so you're less likely to overeat. Overeating has been seen as a trigger postnasal drip. So, load up on healthy fiber from these foods:

- Whole grains such as oatmeal, couscous and brown rice.
- Root vegetables such as sweet potatoes, carrots and beets.
- Green vegetables such as asparagus, broccoli and green beans.
- A bowl of low-fat mixed nuts

Alkaline foods

Foods fall somewhere along the pH scale (an indicator of acid levels). Those that have a low pH are acidic and more likely to cause postnasal drip, throat clearing, mucus or phlegm in the throat, cough, voice crackling, sore throat, sense that the throat may close, feeling of a scratch or tickle in the throat, feeling of a lump in the throat, tight swallowing, food feeling like it is "going down the wrong pipe" and more. Those with higher pH are alkaline and can help offset strong stomach acid.

Alkaline foods include:

- Bananas
- Melons
- Cauliflower
- Fennel
- Nuts

Watery foods

Eating foods that contain a lot of water can dilute and weaken stomach acid. Choose foods such as:

- Celery
- Cucumber
- Lettuce
- Watermelon
- Broth-based soups
- Herbal tea

Milk (see Chapter 11 also)

Does milk help with heartburn? Milk is thought by many to relieve PND. But milk comes in different varieties — whole milk with the full fat, 2% fat, 1% fat and

THE CLEAR THROAT LIFE | 169

skim or nonfat milk. The fat in milk can aggravate postnasal drip, throat clearing, mucus or phlegm in the throat, cough, voice crackling, sore throat, sense that the throat may close, feeling of a scratch or tickle in the throat, feeling of a lump in the throat, tight swallowing, food feeling like it is "going down the wrong pipe" and more.

Nonfat (skim) milk can act as a temporary buffer between the throat lining and pepsin, foodstuff, acid and bile to provide immediate relief of postnasal drip, throat clearing, mucus or phlegm in the throat, cough, voice crackling, sore throat, sense that the throat may close, feeling of a scratch or tickle in the throat, feeling of a lump in the throat, tight swallowing, food feeling like it is "going down the wrong pipe" and more symptoms.

HERE IS A SAMPLE LIST OF "SAFE" FOODS TO EAT WHEN HAVING PND:

Vegetables and non-citrus fruits — Aside from the "bad" foods listed above, nearly all fruits and vegetables help reduce pepsin, foodstuff, acid and bile. They're also low fat, low sugar, and provide fiber and important nutrients. Bananas, melons, broccoli, asparagus, and green beans are low in acid and known to reduce pepsin, foodstuff, acid and bile levels.

Whole grains — High fiber, whole-grains like brown rice, oatmeal, and whole-grain breads help stop symptoms. They are a good source of fiber and may help absorb pepsin, foodstuff, acid and bile, reducing the risk of symptoms.

Lean protein — Low-fat, lean sources of protein may also reduce symptoms of postnasal drip and more. Good choices are chicken, seafood, tofu, and egg whites. The best ways to prepare them are baked, broiled, poached, or grilled.

Beans, peas, and lentils — Along with being good sources of fiber, beans, peas, and lentils also provide protein, vitamins and minerals.

Nuts and seeds — Many nuts and seeds provide fiber and nutrients and may help absorb pepsin, foodstuff, acid and bile. Almonds, peanuts, chia, pomegranate, and flaxseeds are all healthy choices.

Yogurt — Not only is yogurt soothing to an irritated throat, but it provides probiotics that support your digestive tract. It's also good source of protein.

Healthy fats — Fat is a necessary nutrient but eating too many fatty foods can trigger symptoms. Replacing unhealthy fats with unsaturated fats can help. Avocados, olive oil, walnuts, and soy products are good choices for healthy fats.

29

SPECIAL CASES

Apple Cider Vinegar (ACV)

W hile there isn't enough research to prove that drinking apple cider vinegar works for post-nasal drip, throat clearing, mucus or phlegm in the throat, cough, voice crackling, sore throat, sense that the throat may close, feeling of a scratch or tickle in the throat, feeling of a lump in the throat, tight swallowing, food feeling like it is "going down the wrong pipe" and more, many people swear that it helps. However, you should never drink it at full concentration because it's a strong acid that can irritate the throat. We do not recommend it, but those who do put a small amount in warm water and drink it with meals. It seems to have effect on moving food, pepsin & bile along – otherwise called a "prokinetic agent".

Lemon water

Lemon juice is generally considered very acidic, but a small amount of lemon juice mixed with warm water and honey (see chapter 25) has an alkalizing effect that neutralizes stomach contents. Also, honey has natural antioxidants, which protect the health of cells.

Betaine and hypochlorhydria

There are some who subscribe to the thought that post-nasal drip and many throat symptoms are due to an insufficient amount of acid in the stomach, a condition called hypochlorhydria.

Analogously, some believe that taking someone without low acid and giving them medicine for acid will actually make postnasal drip and more symptoms worse. As of this writing, these concepts are theoretical and more research needs to be done. We do not advise using betaine for postnasal drip, throat clearing, mucus or phlegm in the throat, cough, voice crackling, sore throat, sense that the throat may close, feeling of a scratch or tickle in the throat, feeling of a lump in the throat, tight swallowing, food feeling like it is "going down the wrong pipe" and any other throat symptoms.

Bromelain and protein metabolism

Some people are on a "high protein" diet, like athletes. Some experience postnasal drip and more symptoms as part of this diet. Using the supplement called Bromelain or eating foods high in bromelain could help in this circumstance.

"Reflux types"

Some non-medical people are selling products about specific types of reflux (wet, dry, splenic, hepatic, etc.), and they may be on to something. However, the data are currently lacking. **This book is about trying to help the most amount of people and speaking about the experience and "expert opinion" of the patients who have helped me understand the TSL.**

Lung disease

Many patients have a dry cough due to lung conditions. If you have a dry cough without other symptoms on the TSL, the clear throat life pathway may or may not benefit you.

Immune deficiency.

Some patients have a specific immune system condition with recurrent infections. Also, many patients are on fancy / new medicine (often injected) that decreases the body's natural ability to fight infection. In these cases,

174 | MICHAEL KORTBUS, MD

the clear throat life pathway may or may not benefit you.

Tic, or nervous condition

There are some who clear their throat as part of a nervous tic. There are therapies about this that you should discuss with your HCW. In these cases, the clear throat life pathway may or may not benefit you.

Pregnancy

As alluded to in several chapters above, pressure on the throat is a cause for postnasal drip, throat clearing, mucus or phlegm in the throat, cough, voice crackling, sore throat, sense that the throat may close, feeling of a scratch or tickle in the throat, feeling of a lump in the throat, tight swallowing, food feeling like it is "going down the wrong pipe" and more. Pregnancy causes this in many. However, the clear throat life plan should be discussed with your obstetrical team, and hopefully your PND and TSL should be short-lived. For those who are pregnant, the clear throat life pathway may or may not benefit you.

Head and Neck Cancer (HNC)

Otolaryngologists (ENT doctors), physician assistants / associates, nurse practitioners, nurses and other advanced practice providers care deeply about those who have HNC. The growth itself, the surgery for it and /or the radiation for it – as well as possible chemotherapy – can each yield postnasal drip and many more symptoms. In these cases, the clear throat life may or may not benefit you.

Health care visits

If you have postnasal drip, throat clearing, mucus or phlegm in the throat, cough, voice crackling, sore throat, sense that the throat may close, feeling of a scratch or tickle in the throat, feeling of a lump in the throat, tight swallowing, food feeling like it is "going down the wrong pipe" and more of these types of symptoms, you should visit your HCW (health care worker). You may need to see an ENT (ear, nose and throat HCW), a pulmonologist (lung HCW), and or a GI (gastroenterologist HCW). Not everyone has had the "complete work up" for PND – but you should.

Dental Disease

From time to time, there will be a patient with either one specific dental problem (one cavity) or generalized dental disease (excess plaque and tartar) who will have TSL. Many are unable to access dental care so may not improve despite all Clear Throat Life aspects written here.

There could be other special conditions not listed in the clear throat life, as well as special medicines that might be the exact answer for you – be sure to check in with these health care workers.

ENJOY THE CLEAR THROAT LIFE!

EPILOGUE

I appreciate your taking the time to read this book and would hope that you can give a strong 5-star recommendation. I am open to suggestions for the next edition as well!

Recommend it to your friends and use this book as a reference. My prayer is that you have found pearls of great price within it.

ABOUT THE AUTHOR

Dr. Michael Kortbus is & has been a practicing physician and surgeon in the field of ear-nose- and throat (otolaryngology) for two decades in New York, where he practices and resides with his wife and children. He has helped countless people with postnasal drip and throat problems, allergies, sinusitis, and more.

If you are interested in a consultation or coaching with Doctor Kortbus, please visit clearthroatlife.com.

Enjoy the Clear Throat Life!

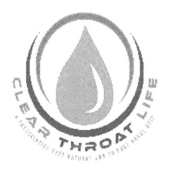